Contents

Acknowledgments

I am so fortunate and grateful for the people and opportunities that have been set in my path. I would like to thank the many people who have contributed to this book in one way or another:

Savka Mladenovich, a teacher who encouraged me to be the Oak Forest High School student council president and gave me my first taste of leadership and love of the microphone in school assemblies.

Lisa Herzig, a dietitian who coached me in my first job as a dietitian at Wild Oats health food store, which set my nontraditional career path in motion.

Dr. Robert Kushner, who mentored me to become a media-savvy, evidenced-based professional and encouraged me to pursue a position as an American Dietetic Association (ADA) spokesperson.

The amazing ADA public relations team (past and present)—Doris Acosta, Tom Ryan, Irene Perconti, Jennifer Starkey, Julia Dombrowski, Liz Spittler, and Lori Ferme—for their tireless support and the countless opportunities they offer to me. Ron Moen, chief executive officer of the ADA, who leads the organization of 67,000 members that I am so proud to represent in television, web, and print media outlets.

Elisa Zied, a fellow ADA spokesperson, for encouraging me to contact her talented literary agent, Stacey Glick.

Stacey Glick of Dystel and Goderich Literary Management, who has stood behind this project since my very first e-mail to her in October 2005 and offered expert advice through the whole proposal and book-writing process.

Carol Svec, the talented writer who helped me organize this project and write a proposal that resulted in multiple publishers knocking on my door.

Doug Seibold, publisher and editor in chief of Agate Publishing in Chicago, who believed in my message and platform even before other publishers.

The talented publishing team at McGraw-Hill who believed in this project: editors Judith McCarthy and Sarah Pelz for holding my hand through this process and editing my work to make it much stronger.

Also thanks to Fiona Sarne, editorial assistant, and Nancy Hall, senior project editor.

My hundreds and hundreds of clients and cooking-class participants who use my flexitarian strategies and advice to live happier and healthier lives. Seeing their effort and success inspires and motivates me to be a dietitian.

Shelley Young, the owner of the Chopping Block Cooking School in Chicago, for giving me the opportunity to teach Healthy in a Hurry flexitarian cooking classes.

Lifetime Television and mylifetime.com, *Fitness* magazine, *All You* magazine, and *Health* magazine for consistently giving me the opportunity to share healthy nutrition messages.

Amy Baltes, a dietitian and friend who let me bounce ideas off of her at midnight when her three kids were asleep and helped me tirelessly with the recipes and grocery lists, even on her birthday.

My three elite girlfriends Tiffany Keller (thanks for the psych advice in the book), Holly Forsyth, and Cathy O'Brien, who let me talk about food and nutrition all the time, get excited about all of my projects, and are there for me even after I fall off the radar for chunks of time.

Susie Lee, a girlfriend and makeup artist who does a fabulous job keeping me looking my best in headshots and encourages me to stay hydrated, use eye cream, and slather on sunscreen for healthy skin.

A special thanks to my girlfriend Kris Genovese. She and I became best of friends a decade ago while eating vegan Greek salads and sunbathing in a kiddie pool in New Mexico. She is the talented designer behind my website dawnjacksonblatner.com and gives me plenty of crazy vegan food ideas to try. I always look forward to the annual batch of vegan chocolate-chip Christmas cookies she bakes for me.

Cecelia and John Gieras, my grandparents. Papa's little porkies (pork sausages) made with love remind me how thankful I am to be a flexitarian rather than a strict vegetarian, and Grandma's openness to try veggie burgers reinforces that flexitarian eating can be embraced by people of all ages.

Herb Jackson IV, my handsome brother, has more character and charisma than anyone I have ever known. I couldn't be more proud of the man he has become. Thanks for tasting my flexitarian food and giving me those encouraging words, "This tastes like fancy restaurant food." I love it when you and Shannon come to cooking class.

Herb and Nance Jackson, my mom and dad, who raised me to believe I could do anything I put my mind to and have always put my happiness before all else. My health-conscious parents, who would rather be bike riding than sitting on the couch, have been great role models for good health, honesty, strong work ethic, and the power of positive mental attitude. Every single day of my life I have felt encouragement, support, and love from them; I thank my lucky stars that I have such amazing people for parents.

Christian, my smart, athletic, and thoughtful stepson, for his understanding and encouragement of my career, even when I am hidden in my office working and miss too many hockey games to count.

Chris, my hot husband and best friend, who gives me daily support, constant encouragement, and unconditional love. When I am swamped with work, he always makes sure I am well hydrated, fed, and loved. He is an honest taste tester of and guinea pig for hundreds of recipes. I am so proud of the flexitarian eater he has become. I fell in love with him over a tofu cutlet he learned to make just for me, and my love for him grows with each passing day.

A final thanks to everyone who is reading this book and allowing me to share the flexitarian approach to a healthier and happier life. I am so excited you've decided to take a proactive role in achieving optimal health. Health is a precious commodity—be good to the body you have and it will be good to you.

Introduction

Flex Effects—Weight Loss, Disease Prevention, and So Much More

I was a closet meat eater, a vegetarian trying not to get caught with a pork chop, beef patty, or chicken sausage in my hand. Now I am a flexitarian and don't have to wear a scarlet letter for eating a little red meat.

I want to be a vegetarian because of the countless health benefits. I also want to enjoy backyard barbecue hamburgers in the summertime, hot dogs at a Cubs baseball game, Grandma's pork roast made with love, my father-in-law's beef chili, Mom's perfectly seasoned steak grilled to perfection by Dad, and Thanksgiving turkey. Oh, and I can't forget the brat-on-a-stick I enjoy with my husband and stepson at the Sheboygan, Wisconsin, annual Brat Days fest. I passionately want to be a vegetarian, but I also want to eat meat on occasion. I and many other people just can't be full-time vegetarians—there are too many appetizing, meaningful meat events in our lives to quit meat cold turkey. The answer is to become a flexible vegetarian—a flexitarian.

I am a *vegetarian* who is *flexible* enough to eat some meat, poultry, and fish—a *flexitarian*. I didn't make this word up. As a matter of fact, it was selected by the American Dialect Society as the Most Useful Word of the Year in 2003. I am not alone in enjoying part-time vegetarian eating—a 2003 study in the *American Journal of Clinical Nutrition* looked at a national sample of more than 13,000 people and found that nearly two out of three vegetarians eat this way. I started talking about flexitarian eating to my clients, family, and friends and found out that so many people already follow this eating style, but there was no guidebook on how to be a healthy flexitarian. So I decided to write the first flexitarian diet book to guide all of the flexible vegetarians out there. Flexitarians can be vegetarian, inclined toward vegetarianism, or just health conscious—you are probably a flexitarian right now and just don't know it!

I have always been intrigued by the power of healthy food—especially plant-based foods. I was born (in March, which is National Nutrition Month) with a loud internal truth or message playing over and over inside of me: "Eating right is the most important thing you can do for yourself." I have always deeply believed that healthy food has the power to heal and make us feel and look our best. We all are put on this earth to contribute something special to one another—my purpose is to excite and motivate people to eat more plants.

With this passion and respect for the power of food, I became a registered dietitian (RD)—a credential I am proud of because RDs are the most trusted and respected food and nutrition experts. As an RD I have closely studied food and nutrition research for more than a decade. One thing remains clear—plants protect people. As a plant grows, it produces a wide variety of natural chemicals called phytochemicals (*phyto* means "plant"). The phytochemicals are the plant's immune system—helping defend it against the scorching sun, wild winds, too little or too much rain, and bothersome bugs. When people eat plants, these phytochemicals protect us against all types of disease.

Eating a plant-based vegetarian diet is the hands-down, smartest thing we can do for our health. On average, vegetarians weigh less than their carnivorous counterparts; have fewer diseases such as heart disease, diabetes, and cancer; and live an average of 3.6 years longer! Based on the science, people would be thinner and healthier if they became vegetarians. But this book is not intended to turn you into a meat-bashing vegetarian who sits at the barbecue with an empty bun—oh no! I want to help you become my kind of vegetarian—the vegetarian who is *flexible* enough to include some red meat, poultry, and fish into your diet: a *flexitarian*. This is a win-win eating plan because you will enjoy the health benefits of vegetarianism without all of the rules and restrictions.

I have taught flexitarian eating to all of the thousands of clients I have counseled over the past ten years, and I have seen my clients lose twenty, fifty, and even eighty pounds. I see health improvements in my clients, such as improved energy levels, self-esteem, arthritis symptoms, blood pressure, and cholesterol, triglyceride, and glucose levels, not to mention weight loss, shrinking waist measurements, and more restful sleep. All of these results were made possible with the flexitarian principles that

I outline in this book. Although clients tell me they immediately start feeling better and love the effects of going Flex, life-changing results are gradual (six to twelve months or more). This isn't a fad diet or a quick fix—by now you know those don't work. You don't want a fad diet—you want lifelong weight loss, overall health and wellness, and improved quality of life. That is what *The Flexitarian Diet* is all about—teaching you a way to live healthier so you can expect results year after year after year.

I have reviewed diet books for magazines and newspapers. Because I critique many new diet books before they even hit the shelves, I know what to look for in a good one—realistic and scientifically sound advice. No quick fixes or junk science. So within the pages of *The Flexitarian Diet* you will find realistic and scientifically sound information. You will find tips, tricks, and strategies for all types of situations and recipes that are tasty and quick.

I know something very special and powerful: plants protect people. *The Flexitarian Diet* presents a realistic and delicious way to eat more plants; this diet will change your life as it has mine and so many others who follow it. I am your liaison between the standard American diet we all enjoy and the healthier, more alternative vegetarian lifestyle. I will show you how to eat more plants without drastically changing how you already are eating and without turning you into a long-haired, crunchy granola hippie. There is no right way to do this—just have fun and experiment. You can incorporate the flexitarian concepts and recipes into your current lifestyle at your own pace—fast or slow.

On Your Mark, Get Set, Flex

I know change is difficult. I hear it every day from my clients. They tell me what market research also shows: most of us like to eat what is familiar to us. Sure, we might try a new chicken dish or a new sandwich, but generally we stick to what we know tastes good and is easy. If you look at the food in your pantry and refrigerator, you'll probably see shelf after shelf of familiar brands. Pasta, bread, snacks, canned soup, breakfast cereal . . . we don't take chances with our food choices. Most of the time, we're too busy to think about it. When I'm having a particularly crazy week (which, to be honest, is most weeks), I like to shop as quickly as possible. I run in, grab the items I need, and dash out. Once, after my grocery store had rearranged all of the items in its aisles, I ran in for some canned tomatoes and wound up frustrated when my favorite brand wasn't on the left bottom shelf of aisle five. I felt disoriented and a little annoyed. I had been running on automatic pilot, but when my routine was disrupted, I had to actually *think*! I was forced to stop, look up and down the aisles, and spend precious time hunting for something that should have been a no-brainer to pick up.

Day to day, most of what we do is routine. We wake up at about the same time, drive on the same roads, do the same chores at home, and perform the same tasks at work. And we eat the same routine comfort foods that we know are quick and tasty. Going on a diet is the mental equivalent of rearranging the shelves—all of our routines become disrupted. We have to think about something as simple as what's for breakfast. As other life problems kick in—stress at work or tensions in the family—the diet is usually abandoned.

I don't want to rearrange your grocery shelves or disrupt your life. *The Flexitarian Diet* builds on what you have already been eating, so you don't have to clear your fridge and cupboards and start over. There is no need to buy hundreds of dollars of special diet foods. The Flexitarian Diet approach is about making changes slowly and gradually so they become part of your routine. As much as you might like an entire nutritional overhaul, too much change is intimidating and frankly impossible for most people to maintain for more than a few weeks. The foundation of my diet philosophy is this: start where you are today and then move just one step closer to your healthier ideal—just one step, one small change at a time.

With the Flexitarian Diet, your starting point doesn't matter. If your diet consists mainly of fast food and sweets, I can help move your diet in a healthier direction without obsessing about every bite. If you already eat well most of the time, I can show you how to add variety to your routine in a way that will give you powerhouse energy. The *flex*ible part of the Flexitarian Diet is that it works for everyone because it fits every life—the life you lead now, not some idealized version of the perfect person we all wish we could be. One change is the seed of a new habit. One change starts a healthy momentum.

The Flexitarian Diet guides you gradually to a casual vegetarian lifestyle that is flexible enough to include all of your favorite foods. This *inclusive* diet does not focus on taking away foods but adds new foods to those you already eat. In this book I give you delicious and quick recipes to taste, weekly meal plans to try, and fitness tips to incorporate into your lifestyle. You can also find more than fifty Flex troubleshooting tips throughout the book to help you save time and problem solve real-life tricky situations.

I teach flexitarian eating in my cooking classes called Health in a Hurry at the Chopping Block Cooking School in Chicago. I have the participants in each class test and rate my recipes (including all of the recipes in this book) on taste and ease of preparation, and I encourage them to give me honest feedback. And let me tell you, they are real, honest people! They will tell it to me straight whether I have a winner or a loser. Of course, I, too, eat these recipes in my everyday life, serve them to my husband and stepson, and bring them to parties for taste tests with family and friends. I even use these flexitarian recipes in articles I write for national magazines such as *Health* and *Fitness* and for my work as the dietitian for Lifetimetv online (mylifetime.com). All the Flexitarian Diet recipes have about five main ingredients, which make shopping and cooking that much easier. The Flexitarian Diet is based on what science has taught, how I live, and what has worked for my thousands of clients.

Flex Benefits

You can follow the Flexitarian Diet at your own pace—if you run out to try most of the Flex recipes, jump into the Flex meal plans with two feet, and dive into the Flex lifestyle strategies, you will get quick weight loss and health results. But don't worry if you decide to take on the Flexitarian Diet slowly and try a new recipe or strategy only once in a while; you can still expect results. That's the beauty of the Flexitarian Diet; this flexible plan bends and molds to your lifestyle instead of you having to twist and contort your life to fit it. And the benefits are amazing.

Weight Loss

Vegetarians have long been regarded as the superstars of dieters. Dozens of scientific studies analyzed in the April 2006 issue of *Nutrition Reviews* showed that people who eat a vegetarian diet weigh about 15 percent less than nonvegetarians. Today, with obesity being a worldwide epidemic, that's a huge difference. Think of it this way—a nonvegetarian woman who weighs 165 pounds could be 25 pounds lighter if she were a vegetarian. It is estimated that about 45 percent of nonvegetarians are overweight, compared with only 6 percent of vegetarians. That's because vegetarian diets are typically lower in total calories, are higher in fiber, and have a lower proportion of calories from fat. The research is clear: if you follow the Flexitarian Diet, you can expect to see a 20-pound average weight loss (15 to 30 pounds) in six to twelve months—and maintain that over the course of your life.

The good news is you don't have to be 100 percent vegetarian to reap the benefits—several studies, including a study published in the 2003 *International Journal of Obesity and Related Metabolic Disorders*, found that even semivegetarians (flexitarians) weigh less than nonvegetarian meat eaters. Not only does weight loss help people fit in smaller pant sizes, but also even a small 5 percent weight loss decreases the risk of chronic disease and positively affects overall health, including the circulatory (heart, veins, and arteries), nervous, respiratory, reproductive, immune, muscular, skeletal, digestive, urinary, endocrine (hormone regulation), and integumentary (hair, skin, and nails) systems.

Improved Heart Health

Studies have confirmed that people who eat a primarily vegetarian diet have a reduced risk of heart disease. Even after just four weeks of eating a flexitarian diet, a study published in the 2005 *Annals of Internal Medicine* found that total cholesterol levels dropped almost 20 points (LDL bad cholesterol dropped almost 15 points). Flexitarians also have lower blood pressure than nonvegetarians—the average systolic pressure (top number) is about 14 points lower and the diastolic pressure (bottom number) is 6 points lower. It is thought that vegetarians have healthier hearts than nonvegetarians because they have lower body weight; their diet has less total and saturated (bad) fat, more fiber, and more fruits and vegetables (which contain heart-smart potassium and magnesium); and they have higher levels of antioxidants such as vitamin C circulating in their blood to protect them against heart disease.

Decreased Risk of Diabetes

A low-fat, plant-based diet decreases your risk of developing diabetes and its complications. Preliminary studies show that people who already have type 2 diabetes maintain better blood glucose control if they switch to a mostly vegetarian diet. Research in *Diabetes Care*, 2006, found that 43 percent of people with diabetes were able to reduce their diabetes medication after following a plant-based diet during a twenty-two-week study.

Decreased Risk of Cancer

Flexitarians also seem to be able to limit their risk of the disease we fear most—cancer. People who eat a semivegetarian diet have about *40 percent less* risk of dying from cancer than people who eat meat. The American Institute for Cancer Research estimates that we could reduce the number of cancer cases by 30 to 40 percent if we all ate a plant-based diet. Researchers believe that a plant-based diet is protective because it is lower in saturated fat (which is found mainly in meat and other animal products such as butter and cheese), higher in fiber, and higher in phytochemicals. Phytochemicals are plant-based compounds able to protect cells, stop the progression of tumor growth, and slow biochemical signs of aging, and they are found only in plant foods such as fruits, vegetables, beans, nuts, and whole-grain foods. A simple apple contains more than a hundred phytochemicals, while cherries, spinach, carrots, bananas, and every other plant contain hundreds of different phytochemicals that all work together to protect us from cancer and all other chronic diseases.

Longer Life Expectancy

Not only do flexitarians live healthier, but they live longer. A 2003 study in the *American Journal of Clinical Nutrition* found that semivegetarians live on average 3.6 years longer than nonvegetarians.

Improved Taste and Fewer Cravings

The Flexitarian Diet exposes you to new, delicious food. Taste is the most important factor in what people eat. You don't have to be a vegetarian to love vegetarian food. Twenty to 25 percent of Americans already eat four or more meatless meals each week. The National Restaurant Association estimates that eight in ten U.S. restaurants offer vegetarian entrées and 60 percent of people often order a vegetarian entrée when dining out. It is important to try new foods because diet monotony leads to ferocious food cravings. A study in *Physiology and Behavior*, 2000, found that a monotonous diet increased cravings for both men and women. *The Flexitarian Diet* will help tame your food cravings by guiding you to try different, convenient, and tasty foods.

Healthy Earth

Our daily activities, such as the amount of electricity we use, how much we drive, what we buy and waste, and even the food choices we make, impact the environment and is called our *carbon footprint*. The lower our carbon footprint, the better it is for Earth's ecosystems, agriculture, and health. Meat and dairy products take more energy and resources to prepare than plant products, so they leave a higher carbon footprint. It is estimated that vegetarian diets emit 42 percent *less* dangerous gas emissions than a typical American diet. This means that the Flexitarian Diet has a low carbon footprint, naturally! Good for you and good for Earth.

Flex Is Great—So What's the Holdup?

With all of the evidence that a semivegetarian diet is the best thing we could do for our bodies—why isn't everyone eating this way? Research shows (and my clients tell me) that there are three main barriers to starting a vegetarian diet: people don't know how to start and think it sounds difficult, they are worried about missing the taste of meat, and they are concerned the diet change could lead to nutrient deficiencies.

The Flexitarian Diet addresses each of these concerns. This book will show you how to easily start eating more satisfying meat-free meals, how to keep meats and treats in your diet so you never feel deprived, and how to make flexitarian choices that will give you optimal nutrition and improve your overall health.

A study of 200 people reported in *The International Journal of Obesity*, 2008, found that only one person in three wanted to follow a vegetarian diet at first, but after a year, those following the vegetarian diet were more likely to still be on their plan than those following a standard diet. Several other research studies have shown similar results—people follow vegetarian eating plans for longer periods of time and report more satisfaction than other types of weight-loss diets. Moral of the story: even if you are nervous about trying this new way of eating—in the end you will be happy that you did!

Instead of rules, I am offering flexibility. Instead of taking foods away, I add new foods to those you already eat. Instead of changing your life to fit the diet, you get to eat in a way that is familiar to you, with the tastes you love most. My mission is to help you undo years of confusing information overload and to show you that it is possible to lose weight and feel great without the usual dietary angst, depression, and upheaval. The Flexitarian Diet is so easy and painless that many of my clients don't believe that it could possibly work—that is, until they finally fit into their skinny pants, or their cholesterol drops below the danger zone, or friends start asking for the name of their plastic surgeon because no one could possibly look that good without professional help.

Everyone deserves a chance to experience success. That's why I developed the Flexitarian Diet, a program that fits every person, every family, and every need. You can try it at your own pace. Take what works for you, and abandon the stuff you hate. The Flexitarian Diet is inclusive—there is room for all your favorite foods, for your family's taste preferences, and for choice. There are no forbidden foods. All you need to do is trust that the system works. Just start by making at least one flexitarian change, and you'll be on the road to a healthier and happier you.

Part One

Getting Started: The Five-by-Five Flex Plan Design

The Flexitarian Diet philosophy is simple but powerful: eat more plants and do the best that you can. Remember that the word *flexitarian* is *flexible + vegetarian*, so this isn't a strict plan outlining good versus bad foods or providing charts with rigid rules about "Eat this but not that." The Flexitarian Diet doesn't judge what you are currently eating; rather, it asks you to include more plant foods and try new things. Keep an open mind (and mouth) when it comes to this plan and you will succeed.

The Flexitarian Diet asks you to put down the paper and pen and put away the measuring cups and food scale—you will neither count calories nor measure out food. Several studies, including a study in the *American Journal of Medicine*, 2005, found that you can lose weight on a vegetarian-type diet without measuring or counting calories. Women in the study lost an average of thirteen pounds just by incorporating more plant foods into their diet. Sure, we will review the importance of being mindful at meals and watching portion sizes, but this is not a diet that will have you calculating every morsel, gram, or crumb that touches your lips. Let this diet be about what foods you *add* to your current routine, not what you will cut, reduce, eliminate, abolish, or omit! The goal is to eat more plants. Do the best you can, and I will show you how I do it and how thousands of my clients have, too . . . using the five Flex components in this book.

The Flex Five

The Flexitarian Diet has five components that will lead you to lose 15 percent of your body weight; prevent diseases such as heart disease, diabetes, and cancer; live longer; and get reenergized to live the life that you want. These five components will guide you to eat and enjoy a balanced, flexible vegetarian diet:

1. Five Flex food groups
2. Five-week Flex meal plan
3. Five-main-ingredient Flex recipes
4. Five Flex fitness factors
5. Five types of FlexLife troubleshooters

Let's look at each of the Flex Five in more detail.

Five Flex Food Groups

Becoming a flexitarian is about adding foods (five Flex food groups to be exact). So often when I tell people I am a flexitarian, they say, "Oh, so you don't eat meat, right?" I guess that is true on a basic level, but the flexitarian lifestyle is not about what you *don't* eat—it is about what you *do* eat! The following five Flex food groups will become your finger-licking favorites:

Flex Food Group 1: Meet the New Meat. When meat is taken out of the equation, people often express a concern about where their necessary protein will come from. Really, protein is found in more foods than you realize—many that you may have been intimidated by or reluctant to try.

I will introduce you to many plant proteins that you will look forward to eating because they not only taste good and are easy to prepare but also make you feel much less heavy than a typical meat-based meal does. I will talk about the myth of meat—how we think we need it despite plenty of other ways to get the same nutritional value.

Many of my clients are surprised to learn that part of the reason people may fail at becoming vegetarian is because meat is a textural flavor. We used to be taught that the tongue could taste four main flavors—sweet, sour, bitter, and salty. Actually, a fifth taste, umami, is a savory taste common in meats, fish, dairy, and some vegetables. When people cut meat out of their diets without replacing the umami taste, they can feel dissatisfied, as though something is missing. It's not the meat, it's the umami. I discuss the importance of umami and how to reduce (not eliminate) meat intake without feeling deprived. (You can even ask my devoted meat-loving husband on this one: you won't miss it.) For this food group, I will help you use the veggie white meat (I try not to use the word *tofu*), beans, lentils, peas, nuts and seeds, and eggs.

Flex Food Group 2: Veg Out and Satisfy Your Fruit Tooth. Because 50 percent of the word *vegetarian* is the word *vegetable*, you have to expect the Flexitarian Diet to have you beef up on your veggies. Studies show that increasing amounts of produce decreases total daily calorie intake without increasing feelings of hunger or deprivation. A study in the *American Journal of Clinical Nutrition*, 1991, found that when participants were encouraged to eat more fruits and vegetables, they consumed 40 percent fewer calories (down from 2,594 to 1,596 calories per day) without increased hunger. I won't just tell you to eat more vegetables—I will give you realistic strategies, show you new tricks, and share great-tasting recipes to naturally rev up your love for veggies. For example, about 25 percent of the population are "supertasters"—people who are extra sensitive to bitter tastes found in foods such as vegetables. I will share three fabulous tricks to help combat the bitter veggie taste. I will also explain how to use a technique called flavor-flavor training to make you *want* to eat your vegetables and actually find yourself asking for seconds!

We are born with a natural love, affinity, and preference for sweet flavors, so as adults we should not deny ourselves sugary satisfaction. Instead of looking to the Keebler Elves to make us cookies or Ben and Jerry to churn a batch of ice cream—a better solution is to reach for fructose, natural sugar found in fruit.

Fruits help give us the sweet taste we desire with the added benefits of vitamins, minerals, antioxidants, and other disease-fighting compounds. Plus, fruit is filling because it has lots of fiber and is about 75 to 95 percent water. (Research has found that foods full of water help keep us feeling full.) I will show you how to front-load your day with fresh fruits to prevent the 3 P.M. sweet tooth and also how to make indulgent, fancy fruit desserts that will have visions of peaches and plums dancing in your head.

Flex Food Group 3: Go with the Grain. Whole grains have three wholesome parts (what I like to call the "trinity of grainy goodness"): bran, germ, and endosperm. These three parts help prevent diseases, such as heart disease, diabetes, obesity, and some types of cancers, such as colon cancer. I will help you find interesting new ways to use whole-grain staples such as whole-grain bread and pasta, oatmeal, popcorn, and brown rice. I will also help you explore (and pronounce) more unusual whole grains such as amaranth, barley, buckwheat, bulgur, kamut, millet, mochi, quinoa, rye, sorghum, spelt, teff, triticale, and wheat berries.

Flex Food Group 4: Dairy Discovery. Dairy's claim to fame (and why it gets its own food group) is its bone-building dynamic duo of calcium and vitamin D. Dairy is also a protein-rich food with potassium, vitamin A, vitamin B_{12}, riboflavin, niacin, and phosphorus. I will lead you on a discovery of all types of dairy foods from traditional low-fat milk and flavorful cheeses to immune-boosting yogurt and kefir (a yogurt-type drink) with billions of healthy bacteria to nondairy alternatives such as soy milk.

Flex Food Group 5: Sugar and Spice (and Everything in Between). This food group is all about the little things that take food from fair to fabulous. I will explore ingredients and condiments that give your recipes extra pop, panache, and pizzazz. I will introduce you to my favorite fresh and dried herbs; teach you what spices are must-haves on your rack; share my favorite salad dressing; explore many sweeteners, such as maple, agave nectar, brown rice, and barley syrups; review first-class condiments such as flaxseeds, non-butter spreads, vinegars, and healthy and flavorful oils (beyond the usual favorites of canola and olive); and even experiment with a little seaweed!

Five-Week Flex Meal Plan

The five-week Flex meal plan organizes all of the recipes into the ultimate flexitarian eating approach. Plus, I give you complete weekly Flex grocery lists to make shopping a snap. You don't have to follow the plan exactly to get health and weight benefits; just remember the goal is progress and not perfection.

I began creating meal plans for my clients after reading a study in the 1996 *International Journal of Obesity and Related Metabolic Disorders* where participants who received meal plans kept off twice as much weight as people who didn't get meal plans. Meal plans work, so I have given you five weeks' worth. The difference between other diet plans and this one is—no surprise—this Flex meal plan is *flexible*! I have designed it to be mix and match. If the barbecue tofu dinner doesn't sound appealing to you—skip it. If you enjoy eating pistachios as a snack every day—do it. Love to start most mornings off with waffles? Eat 'em! Want dark chocolate for an evening snack? Enjoy it!

In total, there are thirty-five breakfast recipes, thirty-five lunches, thirty-five dinners, and thirty-five different snacks. I organize all of the recipes into five weeks, each with seven breakfasts, seven lunches, seven dinners, and seven snack choices. You can swap recipes from different weeks to best meet your needs and preferences. If you want to do the plan exactly as I have outlined, that's fine too.

The meals and snacks can be mixed and matched based on my "*3-4-5*" meal-plan system: breakfast choices are each around *3*00 calories, lunches are *4*00 calories, and dinners are *5*00 calories. (Instead of being as easy as one-two-three, this meal plan is as easy as three-four-five!) The snacks are about 150 calories each, and when you choose two, the day's calories add up to about 1,500—the perfect amount to lose weight without sacrificing satisfaction. The 3-4-5 plan is a good way to evenly spread your calories through the day. About

60 percent of your meal calories come before dinner, which helps control your energy and appetite levels the entire day.

Depending on activity level, gender, height, and weight, you may need slightly more or fewer calories. Women typically need 1,200 to 1,500 calories per day for weight loss, and men may need 1,800 to 2,000. At 1,500 calories per day, the Flex plan is a good place for most people to start. To make it a 1,200-calorie plan, omit the snacks. For an 1,800-calorie plan, double the portion at breakfast. If you are losing too slowly, pay more attention to portions, and if you are losing too fast, add a snack or an extra portion at the meal when you are the hungriest.

Get bored easily when on a diet plan? There are more than 8,000,000 (yes, that is not a misprint: eight million!) different ways you can mix and match these breakfasts, lunches, dinners, and snacks (thanks to my mathematical, genius brother for number crunching the possible meal and snack combos!). Too busy to cook? The plan is designed to be quick and easy so you can sink your teeth into the flavorful meals and snacks even on your most time-crunched days.

Five-Main-Ingredient Flex Recipes

The Flex recipes are the foundation of the Flexitarian Diet. The two goals of the Flex recipes are to help you (1) easily prepare healthy flexitarian foods and (2) enjoy eating healthy flexitarian foods. The recipes average just *five* main ingredients. I tried to keep them around five ingredients because that is the average number of items a person buys at the grocery store to make a quick meal (75 percent of us make same-day dinner decisions and grab our five dinner ingredients off grocery store shelves in less than twenty minutes). For most of us, meals take about thirty-four minutes to prepare—so these recipes are designed with our need for speed in mind! The meals are so fast that I would call it "meal assembly" rather than really cooking.

The Flex recipes take healthy, quick, and convenient ingredients, such as canned beans, from blah to ta-dah. I developed these recipes while experimenting in my kitchen—the recipes in this book are all things I love to eat. I make these meals all week long and even for special occasions. I also use these recipes in the magazine articles I write and the cooking classes I teach. Even if you see a recipe with ingredients you are reluctant to eat or think you don't like—try it! In each of my cooking classes, I have at least one class participant who begins class by bean bashing—announcing how much he or she loathes beans—only to become a bean believer after tasting the recipes. Tasting is believing.

Of course, you won't like every recipe and meal idea here. So I include Flex Swap tips for ingredients in some recipes for variations that may better suit your taste preferences or to help you use other ingredients you may have on hand in your kitchen. In addition to the recipes, I'll give you a must-have list of Flex fridge, pantry, and spice rack staples, and a checklist of essential Flex kitchen tools that any healthy, efficient kitchen should keep stocked. Just trying one of the Flex recipes is the first step to becoming a leaner, healthier, and more energetic you.

The recipes are organized and grouped into a five-week meal plan. Please remember you don't have to do the full five-week Flex meal plan—you can just try a recipe here and there. Becoming flexitarian needs to happen on your own timeline—making lifestyle changes should be somewhat challenging but shouldn't be frustrating or overwhelming. In the end, you should have fun being flexible and enjoy your flexitarian food while getting fabulous results—whether you do it one Flex recipe at a time, try one week's worth of Flex meals, or embark on the full five-week Flex meal plan. In addition to trying the meal plans and recipes, the Flexitarian Diet is a *lifestyle*, so the next part of the book focuses on facets of your fitness life.

Five Flex Fitness Factors

I know this isn't news to anyone: for any weight-loss diet or healthy-living plan to work long-term, you need to exercise. In 2007, the American College of Sports Medicine and the American Heart Association clearly outlined minimum exercise recommendations: in addition to light activities of daily living, adults should moderately exercise for thirty minutes, five days per week (or intensely exercise for twenty minutes, three times per week), and strength train at least two days per week.

A variety of barriers can prevent starting and sticking with an exercise program. In this part we will first emphasize the key mantra to maintaining a flexitarian exercise program: "Anything is better than nothing." I will outline how to look at the world as your gym, use start-up strategies, maintain motivation, try tools of the trade, and beat exercise barriers.

Five Types of FlexLife Troubleshooters

The five types of FlexLife troubleshooters are valuable tips to help you overcome the hurdles of healthy changes and weight loss. They are diet-survival strategies for the challenges life can throw at you. There are more than fifty troubleshooters in all, so you should find information and inspiration from one of five different categories (each with its own eye-catching icon) on just about any page:

FlexLife Troubleshooter 1: Fact Stack
Fact Stack troubleshooters answer frequently asked questions about flexitarianism, dieting, and weight loss.

FlexLife Troubleshooter 2: Time Crunch
Time Crunch troubleshooters make healthy changes speedy and efficient.

FlexLife Troubleshooter 3: Craving Control
Craving Control troubleshooters are tips to tame even your most ferocious cravings and curb emotional eating.

FlexLife Troubleshooter 4: Out and About

Out and About troubleshooters cover common diet roadblocks and challenges at restaurants, at parties, and while traveling.

FlexLife Troubleshooter 5: Feeling Good

Feeling Good troubleshooters focus on mental wellness and healthy attitude adjustments.

I hope it is obvious that I have all your diet needs covered. This is about more than just information—all the facts in the world won't help you lose weight. Beyond the facts, I offer you quick recipes, realistic fitness tips, and workable strategies to overcome barriers, obstacles, life events, and personal foibles that get in the way of weight loss and living the healthy life you want. With the Flexitarian Diet, there is no way to fail . . . but there are five-by-five paths to success.

Setting the Right Flex Goal

I know that you probably had a certain set of goals in mind when you bought this book. In my practice, I've heard them all, including some that are wildly unrealistic. Clients come to see me fully expecting to lose fifty pounds in two months, to whittle themselves down to a size 2, or to get off insulin treatment for type 2 diabetes in time for Super Bowl Sunday. The Flexitarian Diet will help you lose weight, reduce your size, and gain control over your nutrition-related health problems, but I want you to lose your attachment to size distinctions and artificial deadlines. The truth is, human beings don't respond well to stress. Some people boomerang and end up gaining weight as their deadline approaches and they realize they won't accomplish what they set out to do. Others will lose weight in time for that special occasion but then gain it all back again once life returns to normal. Weight loss should not be a race or a contest. Set yourself free by tossing aside the dates and numbers—you'll feel so much better without all that added pressure.

Let's set you up with a different kind of goal. Rather than aiming for a particular weight or size, invest your energies in thinking about getting healthy, one small change per day. We each make hundreds of decisions about our health each day. Research shows we make 226.7 decisions about food daily—even just one change (a change of 0.5 percent) can positively affect the quality of our life and overall health. Commit to making just one flexitarian change, no matter how big or small, and in making that change you can consider yourself successful. If you want to make more than one flexitarian change, great. But one small change per day is a healthy start.

Feeling Good

Don't consider this a diet. Consider this a *nondiet*-lifestyle approach to get healthy and lose weight. Dieters have lower body satisfaction as well as a lower quality of life than nondieters.

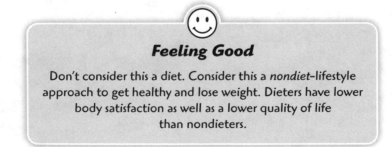

You can choose to make any change you want. For example, try a quick Flex breakfast instead of skipping the most important meal of the day, swap your typical 3 P.M. vending machine snack with a nutritious Flex snack, do a Flex fitness activity, or practice a Flex restaurant strategy. There are thousands of realistic changes throughout this book—your goal is to focus on at least one each day. You will wake up one morning to find you have inched your way to living a wildly healthy Flex lifestyle—one change at a time.

When I tell this to my clients, they are skeptical at first. No one ever believes that one change will fix anything, let alone a problem as stubborn as weight. They are accustomed to hearing—from their doctors, media reports, or other diet books—that almost everything they have been doing is wrong. So when I tell them that most of what they are doing is fine and making one change will launch them to a new and improved version of themselves, they think I'm crazy. But they try it. After a month, nearly everyone is a Flex convert. I have seen it with friends, family members, cooking-class participants, and my clients. Commit to making at least one Flex change each day—it is that easy. Small changes make a big difference over time.

Fact Stack

Weigh yourself regularly. Daily or weekly weigh-ins help you stay mindful of your goals. If you don't like scales, pick a pair of nonelastic pants to gauge your weight fluctuations.

Your FlexScore: How Flex Are You?

Healthy eating is a journey. I want to help you get healthier one step at a time. Where are you right now on the Flex eating journey? Take the following quiz to find out your FlexScore. Are you a beginner, advanced, or expert flexitarian? As you start making Flexitarian Diet changes, retake the test to see your FlexScore improve.

What's Your FlexScore?

For each of the following statements, put a number from 1 to 4 that indicates how you feel about the statement: 1 = strongly disagree, 2 = disagree, 3 = agree, and 4 = strongly agree.

1. I eat at least 2½ cups of vegetables each day. ____
2. I eat at least 2 cups of fruit each day. ____
3. I try a new produce item or new recipe using produce every week. ____
4. When I eat or prepare desserts, I try to incorporate fresh fruit. ____
5. My grocery cart almost always is filled with 50 percent produce. ____
6. I consume orange or green fruits and vegetables most days. ____
7. I confidently can convert a recipe with beef, pork, chicken, or turkey into a bean-based vegetarian dish. ____
8. I eat 1 cup or more of beans or a bean-based dish most days. ____
9. I am confident in preparing tofu and tempeh. ____

10. If I don't eat fish at least twice a week (12 ounces per week), I consume 1 to 2 tablespoons of ground flaxseed or flaxseed oil daily. _____

11. I check labels to see that the ingredients on my cereal, bread, and pasta use the term *100 percent whole grain.* _____

12. I regularly eat and prepare whole grains such as barley, corn, millet, oat, quinoa, brown rice, and bulgur. _____

13. I consume two to three servings (16–24 ounces) of dairy or dairy alternatives each day. _____

14. I limit the amount of cheese I eat and opt for healthier fats for flavor, such as avocado, olive oil, nuts, and seeds. _____

15. I typically use herbs and spices other than just salt and pepper to season my food. _____

16. I drink 9 to 12 glasses (72–96 ounces) of primarily water and other low-calorie beverages (such as tea and coffee) per day. _____

17. I eat three meals a day on a regular schedule. _____

18. I am calorie conscious: my breakfast is around 300 calories, lunch is 400 calories, and dinner is 500 calories (more calories are necessary for very active women and men). _____

19. I eat vegetarian breakfasts (i.e., rarely eat bacon or sausage). _____

20. I eat vegetarian lunches (i.e., rarely eat lunch meat). _____

21. I have two snacks a day (each around 150 calories). _____

22. I usually ask myself if I am physically hungry before I eat a snack. ____

23. I do moderate aerobic exercise thirty minutes a day, five days a week. ____

24. I engage in weight training exercise at least two times per week. ____

25. I feel my daily stress is at an optimal level (I feel excited and alive without feeling overwhelmed). ____

26. I keep my home stocked with healthy choices, and I remove tempting junk foods. ____

27. I keep my work environment stocked with healthy choices, and I remove tempting junk foods (if you work at home, use the same answer as for question 26). ____

28. When I dine out, I primarily order vegetarian options. ____

29. If a meaningful social situation or interesting food experience included a beef, pork, chicken, or turkey item, I would eat and enjoy it. ____

30. I am eating foods I enjoy and don't feel like I am on a diet. ____

Add up Your Total FlexScore

If you scored 30 to 60 points: You are a *Beginner Flexitarian*. Welcome! I will expose you to a whole new world of eating foods you enjoy while losing weight and feeling great. Make small and gradual changes so you don't feel overwhelmed or frustrated. Allow yourself to have fun while exploring all that the flexitarian lifestyle has to offer.

If you scored 61 to 91 points: You are an *Advanced Flexitarian*. You already have many healthy Flex behaviors and should be proud of yourself! Continue trying new Flex foods, recipes, and lifestyle tips. With more time and practice you will find yourself reaping maximum benefits from your flexitarian lifestyle.

If you scored 92 to 120 points: Congratulations, you are a seasoned *Expert Flexitarian* and have incorporated lifestyle changes to help you live an extraordinary life. Continue making small healthy changes to your current routine. Use new recipes, push yourself to eat more variety, and try new Flex foods and fitness activities. Keep your motivation high by surrounding yourself with healthy people and thoughts. Talk to other people who are health conscious, and read health and wellness books, magazines, newsletters, and websites. Get involved in healthy activities such as 5K benefit walks or runs, dance classes, tennis lessons, meditation groups, or healthy cooking classes.

Remember, life is dynamic and ever changing. We have to bend and be flexible to withstand the winds of change. At some points in your life you may be able to take on more or less of the Flexitarian Diet. Take the quiz periodically to see where you are on the Flex journey. No matter what your FlexScore is, commit to at least one Flex change (big or small) each day and you will be a Flex success!

Fact Stack

Going Flex Goals

Beginner Flexitarian: Two meatless days per week (26 ounces of meat or poultry per week)

Advanced Flexitarian: Three to four meatless days per week (18 ounces of meat or poultry per week)

Expert Flexitarian: Five or more meatless days per week (9 ounces of meat or poultry per week)

Note: If you choose to eat fish, eat about 12 ounces of a variety of fish per week.

Part Two

Five Flex Food Groups

Becoming a flexitarian is about *adding* foods—the five Flex food groups to be exact—not just taking out meat and other animal foods. In this part of the book, you will become an expert on the five Flex food groups:

Group 1: Meet the new meat
Group 2: Veg out and satisfy your fruit tooth
Group 3: Go with the grain
Group 4: Dairy discovery
Group 5: Sugar and spice (and everything in between)

As you read through the different Flex food groups, I will share personal tips to help you successfully add more Flex foods to your current diet routine. Then you can flip to Part Three, the five-week Flex meal plan, for all of the five-main-ingredient Flex recipes.

Fact Stack

Use the power of one. You don't need to become a completely different person overnight and make multiple changes all at once. List all of the healthy changes you want to make and then pick just *one*. One single change has the momentum for making other healthy changes.

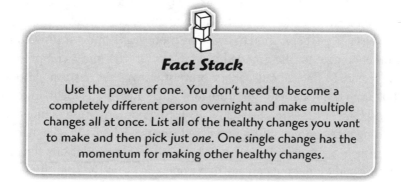

Flex Food Group 1: Meet the New Meat

Let me introduce you to the three basic Flex "meats": legumes (e.g., beans, peas, and lentils), nuts, and seeds. This food group is your most concentrated protein source. The Flex Diet focuses on *plant* proteins, while the standard American diet gets most of its protein from animal proteins such as chicken, turkey, fish, shellfish, pork, beef, cheese, and eggs. Remember, I am not trying to make you turn your back on your lifelong meat buddies, but the Flexitarian Diet is trying to get you to mingle with and befriend the plant-based protein foods. Make new meat friends, and keep the old.

Many people mistakenly believe a common meat myth that you can't get a healthy amount of protein from a vegetarian diet. Not true: the Institute of Medicine of the National Academies recommends that 10 to 35 percent of our calories come from protein. If someone is eating 1,500 to 2,000 calories per day, that translates to a healthy protein range of 45 to 150 grams per day (15 to 50 grams of protein per meal). This easily can be achieved with Flex proteins. For example, cereal with *soy milk* topped with *nuts* and berries for breakfast + 1½ cups of *black bean* soup with a salad and whole-grain roll for lunch + an apple with *peanut butter* for a snack + a barbecue *veggie burger* with sweet potato fries at dinner totals 60 grams of protein, which easily meets the daily protein requirement. Another myth is that vegetarians have to combine certain plant proteins at each meal to make a complete or quality protein. Although that was the thought in the 1970s, we now know that as long as you eat a variety of plant foods throughout the day, you do not need to combine them in any specific way.

Need a little inspiration to try some more veggie meats? How about protection against the dreaded *c* word: *cancer*? The most comprehensive report to date about cancer prevention was released in October 2007 from the American Institute for Cancer Research (AICR) and the World Cancer Research Fund (WCRF). This rigorous study found that limiting meat and avoiding processed meats such as sausage, bacon, and lunch meat was one of their top-ten recommendations for preventing and managing cancer. They concluded that the goal should be eating 18 ounces of red meat *per week* or less and that each additional 1.7 ounces consumed increases cancer risk by 15 percent. The report recommends avoiding processed meat (since it is high in sodium and chemicals called nitrates) altogether because every 1.7 ounces consumed per day increases risk of colon cancer by 21 percent.

Flex meats are primarily plant-based, powerful disease *fighters*. A good rule of thumb is that 25 percent of your grocery cart and 25 percent of your meals should come from this group. You don't have to measure precisely—you can eyeball it. I will walk you through how to add my favorite Flex proteins painlessly and tastefully into your current diet. I will tell you about the taste and texture and give you tips and tricks for shopping and preparing the following Flex meats:

Legumes (beans, peas, lentils)
Veggie white meat—tofu—and its cousin tempeh
Great fakes (soybean-based foods such as veggie burgers, sausages, and corn dogs)
Nuts and seeds
Eggcellent eggs

Love Those Legumes

Beans and all of those lovely legumes such as peas and lentils have a special place in my heart and a prominent place in my pantry. They are low in calories and fat, and they are rich in protein, fiber, folate, iron, potassium, selenium, magnesium, and zinc—not to mention that they are brimming with other health-promoting, disease-fighting compounds such as protease inhibitors, saponins, phytosterols, lectins, and oligosaccharides. Research published in the *Journal of Agriculture Food Chemistry*, 2004, found serving per serving, beans have more disease-fighting antioxidants than almost all other fruits and vegetables. High-antioxidant foods are particularly powerful for fighting cancer, heart disease, and aging.

Beans, peas, and lentils are the only foods that the U.S. Department of Agriculture allows to be officially in two food groups. They are considered a *meat* because they are protein rich, and because they are vitamin rich, they are also considered a *vegetable*. Aim to eat at least 3 cups each week—and with the quick and tasty Flex recipes in this book, those 3-plus cups have never "bean" so delicious! You can also take your own recipes and make them more flexitarian by substituting ¼ *cup of cooked beans, peas, or lentils for every 1 ounce of meat*; a ¼ cup of cooked beans = 60 calories, 0 grams fat, 4 grams fiber, 4 grams protein; and 1 ounce of broiled lean beef = 60 calories, 2 grams fat, 0 grams fiber, 8 grams protein. See the Bean Math Flex Box to find out about how to add up your beans.

You can make legumes from scratch, but I prefer and teach people to use canned because they are just so convenient. Canned foods usually contain salt, so rinse for about forty seconds and drain to decrease the sodium by about 40 percent. If you would like to try to cook your own legumes from scratch, see the Flex Box Sort, Soak, and Simmer Your Beans (on page 24) for basic cooking guidelines. The many different varieties of legumes all have different tastes and textures. The following is a list of my favorite legumes:

Black beans

Taste and texture: Rich, earthy, and soft

Tips and tricks: Buy plenty of these—they are one of my favorites. Black beans are so versatile they can even be hidden in your favorite brownie recipe. Just rinse, drain, and puree one 15-ounce can of black beans. Stir them with your favorite box of brownie mix (you don't need to add any other ingredients). Bake according to the box instructions.

Cannellini beans

Taste and texture: Meaty and smooth

Tips and tricks: They are also called "white kidney beans" and taste great in anything Italian. I also love them in my guacamole recipe (see Index).

FLEX BOX

Bean Math

15-ounce can of beans, rinsed and drained = 1½ cups

One pound of beans = 2 cups dry = 6 cups cooked

Edamame (green, immature soybeans)

Taste and texture: Sweet and slightly crunchy

Tips and tricks: These are not canned; usually they are found in the frozen section. You can get them in the pod or shelled. For a snack, I get edamame in the pod, warm them in the microwave, and add a sprinkle of salt. You don't eat the green, fuzzy pod that they come in—just the beans inside. If I plan to use them in a recipe, I get them shelled (out of the pod).

Garbanzo beans

Taste and texture: Nutty flavor and solid texture

Tips and tricks: They are also called "chickpeas" and are the traditional bean used in hummus recipes. You can toss these whole into recipes or chop them for a totally different texture.

Great Northern beans

Taste and texture: Delicate flavor, tender, and moist

Tips and tricks: After they are rinsed and drained, they puree into a very smooth texture that is perfect for making dips. I use them in many soup recipes because when I partially puree the finished soup, the beans make it thicker and creamier.

Kidney beans

Taste and texture: Subtly sweet and firm

Tips and tricks: You can find light or dark varieties that taste similar, so just choose the color you prefer.

Lentils

Taste and texture: Earthy and soft

Tips and tricks: I buy canned, but if you want to make them from scratch, purchase lentils dry in a bag. Dry lentils take less time to prepare than other beans, because they don't require soaking ahead of time.

Lima beans

Taste and texture: Baby lima beans are green, firm, and plump. Fordhook lima beans are white, much larger, and are more buttery and creamy.

Tips and tricks: Two main varieties of lima beans are available—baby and Fordhook. Since the taste and texture of the two are quite different, be sure to check labels for the specific variety of lima bean. Fordhook lima beans are also called "butter beans." Butter beans are my favorite bean because they are huge, tender, and creamy.

Navy beans

Taste and texture: Mild and plump

Tips and tricks: I get plain, canned navy beans, but navy beans are used in canned baked-bean recipes, too. Canned vegetarian baked beans are delicious, but keep portions to ½ cup because the sodium and calories can add up fast if you eat more.

Peas

Taste and texture: Sweet and tender

Tips and tricks: You can get *dried* split peas in a bag, and they take about 30 minutes of simmering in water to make them soft and tender. My favorite is *frozen* garden peas because after a quick thaw in the microwave or a pan they are ready to eat.

Pinto beans

Taste and texture: Meaty and tender

Tips and tricks: In addition to plain pinto beans in a can, canned refried bean recipes commonly use pinto beans. Stock up on plain pintos and *low-fat or vegetarian* refried beans (which means lard free)—they are easy, affordable, and healthy for all types of Mexican-style recipes.

Fend off Flatulence. Flatulence, gas, toots—whatever you call it—beans are notorious for causing abdominal distention. The natural sugars in beans (called oligosaccharides) are hard for us to digest, so healthy bacteria in our intestines help out. As the bacteria digest these sugars, they let out gas. Flatulence is a major reason why people shy away from beans and other legumes in their diet. Don't be bashful about eating more beans—here are three easy steps to help prevent bean bloat (or gassiness caused by any food):

1. **Baby bean steps.** If you aren't used to eating beans, give your body time to adjust. Add beans to your diet gradually—start with 2 to 4 tablespoons at a time and work your way up to a ½-cup serving or more.
2. **Chew.** Digestion begins in your mouth with the help of enzymes in saliva. Chewing food improves digestion so intestinal bacteria have less work to do and in turn produce less gas.
3. **Try an enzyme helper.** You can purchase over-the-counter enzymes that work to help your digestion. Enzymes (brands such as Beano) can be purchased at grocery stores and drugstores and are taken with your meal to help prevent digestive discomfort.

Veggie White Meat and Its Cousin

Veggie white meat can be marinated, broiled, sautéed, or grilled like chicken breast. It can be mashed, blended, whipped, crumbled, simmered, and steamed. It can be made sweet or spicy. It can be baked in a casserole to give the consistency of cheese or stirred into sauces with the creamy consistency of sour cream. This culinary chameleon is *tofu*. Tofu is made from soybeans and can be one of the most versatile Flex meats in your kitchen. However, many assume that they don't like tofu just because of its name—we crinkle up our noses at just hearing the words *tofu* and *soy*.

The reluctance to try soy foods is truly an issue of mind over matter or, more accurately, mind over taste buds. The names soy and tofu conjure up unpleasant judgment, so let's just toss the word *tofu* and start calling it *veggie white meat*. Tofu's cousin is tempeh. Tempeh is also made from soybeans, but the soybeans are fermented. Many foods we love are fermented like wine, yogurt, cheese, and pickles. During the processing of tempeh, the soybeans also can be mixed with rice, sesame seeds, or other grains and nuts for different flavors. The sturdy texture of tempeh makes it a fantastic stand-in for meat.

Veggie white meat: tofu

Taste and texture: Veggie white meat (tofu) is made by soaking soybeans, extracting the milk, and then adding a compound to curd the milk. Depending on the curdling compounds used, you

FLEX BOX

Sort, Soak, and Simmer Your Beans

Step one: *Sort* and clean. Rinse them under water (I like to put the beans in a glass cake pan with water), and discard any pebbles or shriveled beans.

Step two: *Soak*. There are two ways:

- Slow soak: In a large pot, cover 1 pound (2 cups) dry beans with 8 cups of water. Let beans sit covered in the refrigerator for 8 hours or overnight. Drain water. Fill with fresh water, bring to a boil, and turn down to a simmer.
- Speedy soak: In a large pot, cover 1 pound (2 cups) dry beans with 8 cups of water. Boil beans for about 5 minutes. Take off of heat, and let beans sit covered in refrigerator for 2–4 hours. Drain water. Fill with fresh water, bring to a boil, and turn down to a simmer.

Step three: *Simmer*—beans are done when they can be easily mashed between your fingers or with a fork. Here are approximate simmering times:

Black	1½ hours
Garbanzo	3 hours
Great Northern	2 hours
Kidney	1½ hours
Lima	1½ hours
Navy	2½ hours
Pinto	2½ hours

NOTE: Peas and lentils don't need to be soaked. Simmer for about 30–60 minutes (until tender).

get different textures—and texture is everything when it comes to eating veggie white meat! Some textures are firm and hold their shape well for grilling and stir-fries, some are so soft that they blend into a sour-cream-like texture for dips and smooth-

Fact Stack

Enjoy meals for twenty-nine minutes. Eating slowly can reduce your intake by 70 calories per meal, which translates into a savings of more than 200 calories per day.

ies, and some are in between, such as a ricotta-cheese texture for lasagna. It really is an amazing food that takes on the taste and flavor of whatever you are cooking.

Tips and tricks: Try to choose the "light" versions when available, for one to two times fewer calories and two to three times less fat. The following tofu tutorial can help you choose the right veggie white meat texture for your recipes:

FLEX BOX

Tofu Tutorial

Read the front of each tofu package for the following words:

- **Silken:** Found in 16-ounce water-filled tubs or 12-ounce aseptic packages. Silken tofu blends into a silky smooth, puddinglike texture. Great for puddings, dips, and smoothies, but *not* for stir-fries.
- **Soft, firm, extra firm:** Found in 16-ounce water-filled tubs. *Soft* tofu has a high water content, so it is tender and smooth, which is good for blending into soups, pies, and dressings (similar to silken tofu but a little heftier in texture). *Firm* has a medium amount of water so it is somewhere between a smooth and solid texture, which is good for mashing into a scrambled-egg-like texture or ricotta-cheese-like texture for lasagna. *Extra firm* has a low water content, so it is more solid and keeps its shape, which is perfect for stir-fries or grilling like a chicken-breast cutlet.

continiued

FLEX BOX

Tofu Tutorial (continued)

- **Baked marinated tofu:** Found in shrink wrap without water and usually preseasoned or flavored. Baked marinated tofu has a firm texture and keeps its shape well. Since it is usually preseasoned and flavorful, you can just chop and toss it into salads, pitas, or stir-fries, or slice it into cutlets to throw directly on the grill.

Once you purchase the right tofu texture, here are my pressing and freezing tips for using all types of tofu except silken:

- **Press:** Before using tofu, it is a good idea to *press* it to get the excess water out. This allows the tofu to be firmer and better able to absorb the flavors of cooking. Put tofu between two towels, and press firmly with your hands. Or my preferred method is to stack heavy plates or pans on top of the towel-wrapped tofu for ten minutes or more.
- **Freeze:** If you open a pack and have extra tofu or you have tofu in the fridge and you aren't going to use it by the expiration date, *freeze* it. First press it as previously described; then cut it into bite-size pieces or thin, rectangular shapes and place them in plastic bags. Storing tofu in the freezer does magical things to the texture—it becomes more firm, tough, and chickenlike. It can keep in the freezer for up to six months. It will become yellow in the freezer, but it will turn back to white after you throw it into the dish you are cooking or thaw it in the microwave.

Note that there is no need to press or freeze silken tofu. You just take it out of the package and blend (I use a hand blender) until it is silky smooth. It is used in recipes for dips, smoothies, and puddings. I also use ¼ cup pureed silken tofu in place of one egg in many recipes.

Tempeh

Taste and texture: Tempeh is made from fermented soybeans. It has a fantastic firm and meaty texture.

Fact Stack

You can also read the ingredient list on the package as a tip-off of just how firm your tofu will be. Look at the first ingredients:

• • •

Nigari (magnesium or calcium chloride) indicates the tofu is usually most firm.

• • •

Gypsum (calcium sulfate) indicates the tofu is usually middle-of-the-road firm.

• • •

GDL, or gluconolactone (silken tofu), indicates the tofu is the least firm and blends to a silky smooth consistency.

Tips and tricks: Tempeh comes in long, thin rectangular packages in the refrigerator section of many grocery stores. A popular brand is LightLife. A 4-ounce portion of tempeh has about the same amount of protein and twelve times the fiber as 4 ounces of chicken.

My first experience using tempeh was to try and re-create the McDonald's McRib sandwich—a hearty, barbecue rib sandwich with grilled onions and pickles. Tempeh's texture is the perfect stand-in for my version, which has about five times less saturated fat and 200 fewer calories than the original (you can try the McRib-like recipe on page 195). Crumble tempeh into your favorite chili recipe instead of ground beef or turkey—it is one of the most popular things my cooking-class participants try at home because it is so delicious! Even my meat-loving brother enjoys it, which really says it all.

Try tempeh as a high-protein, crunchy crouton alternative. Preheat the oven to 400°F. Cut the tempeh into half-inch cubes, and toss with lime juice, sesame oil, and minced garlic. Bake on a cookie sheet for thirty minutes until crunchy and toss on top of salad.

Fact Stack

Eat as a family, not family-style. Keep food (except for vegetables) in the kitchen and not directly on the table to help prevent double and triple helpings.

Fake It: Soy Substitutes

There are many veggie versions of meaty products we crave, such as veggie burgers, veggie crumbles (to take the place of ground meat), veggie sausages, veggie chicken strips and patties, and even veggie lunch meats. Some popular brands include Morningstar Farms, Gardenburger, Yves, and Boca. These products tend to have fewer calories, more fiber, and much less artery-clogging saturated fat and cholesterol than their meat counterparts, but you do have to watch their sodium levels. Aim to buy products with less than 500 milligrams of sodium per serving. I particularly like these products because they can be heated quickly in a microwave, toaster oven, or skillet for fast, flavorful meals in minutes.

- **Taste and texture:** It can take some time and patience to find the brands and products that really best "meat" your taste and texture preferences and expectations. These products are more processed, so don't rely on them 100 percent to take the place of meat in your diet.
- **Tips and tricks:** Check two places for these veggie versions: the frozen foods section and the produce section. Read labels for 500 milligrams of sodium or less per serving. Have patience, and try different products until you find those you like the most.

Go Nuts and Seeds

Research studies have found that eating 1 ounce of nuts about five times a week decreases the risk of heart disease by 30 percent. Seeds such as pumpkin, sunflower, flax, and sesame also have heart-smart fats and contribute plant protein to our diets. Variety is important within this nut and seed group because they all have slightly different claims to fame. Almonds and sunflower seeds have the highest vita-

Fact Stack

Try wheat meat. Seitan (pronounced SAY-tahn) is a meat substitute made from wheat gluten. It has a remarkably meaty texture and has about 100 calories per serving, little to no fat, and 18 grams of protein. It can be found in the refrigerated section of health food stores.

min E content, walnuts and flaxseeds have omega-3 fatty acids, pumpkin seeds have the most zinc, and brazil nuts outshine the rest in their selenium content.

- **Taste and texture:** All nuts and seeds have a common crunch but differ greatly in tastes and textures. Nutritionally, nuts and seeds are all rich in heart-healthy unsaturated fats and protein, but only seven of them—almonds, hazelnuts, pecans, peanuts, pine nuts, pistachios, and walnuts—have the U.S. Department of Agriculture's health-claim stamp that they may reduce the risk of heart disease. (Peanuts are technically legumes, not nuts. Since they have the heart-healthy properties of other nuts, most of the time they are just lumped into the nut family.) Other nuts such as brazil, cashew, and macadamia are still healthy but have a little more saturated fat than the others.
- **Tips and tricks:** Nuts and seeds are usually found in at least three places: in the produce section, in the baking aisle, and near the popcorn, candy, and chips. Compare price per ounce to determine where you can get the best deal. Buy them unsalted, or compromise by buying one bag unsalted and one bag salted and mixing them to get a 50 percent salt version. Both roasted and raw nuts give you heart-healthy fats, but raw nuts and seeds last longer and are less likely to have added fats and flavors than the roasted varieties.

Don't forget all the delicious nut and seed butters available, such as peanut butter, almond butter, sunflower seed butter, soynut butter,

FLEX BOX

Nut Ounce Count

1 ounce =	24 almonds
	7 Brazil nuts
	18 cashews
	11 macadamias
	28 peanuts
	20 pecans (halves)
	157 pine nuts
	49 pistachios
	14 walnuts (halves)

and sesame seed butter (called tahini and used in hummus recipes). Opt for natural peanut butter. It has more peanut flavor than processed versions, so you can use less—which is good because almost all types of peanut and other nut and seed butters have 100 calories per just 1 tablespoon.

Nuts are high in healthy fats, which also makes them high in calories. The perfect daily amount is 1 ounce. See the Flex Box Nut Ounce Count to learn how many nuts equals 1 ounce. Even though they are high in calories, research has shown that nuts make you feel more satisfied than other snacks and that nut eaters tend to have lower body weights. I use nuts in many recipes for their protein-packed, heart-smart crunch.

Eggcellent

Whole eggs provide vitamins and minerals for brain health, bones, and vision, such as selenium, choline, riboflavin, phosphorus, folate, vitamin D, lutein, and zeaxanthin. Egg yolks have more vitamins and minerals than the whites, but they also have more calories, fat, and cholesterol. What to do? Compromise by using 1 whole egg + 2 egg whites in recipes instead of 2 whole eggs.

- **Taste and texture:** Eggs are quite versatile and take on just about any flavor; they can be used at breakfast, lunch, or dinner.

- **Tips and tricks:** I tend to buy organic, omega-3-enriched eggs. Eggs labeled "organic" by the U.S. Department of Agriculture (USDA) must come from chickens that are fed organic feed without antibiotics or growth hormones and are given access to the outdoors. It doesn't matter if the eggs are brown or white—that is due to different breeds of hens and doesn't impact the nutritional value of the eggs. For an extra boost of omega-3 (which is especially important for non-fish-eating vegetarians), buy omega-3-fortified eggs, which are typically produced by feeding chickens a higher omega-3 fatty acid diet. Each egg has the omega-3 equivalent to that of about 1 tablespoon of fish. Egg substitutes are low in calories, fat, and cholesterol because they are primarily egg whites, but they also are missing all the vitamins and minerals the yolk provides. Mix one whole egg with an egg substitute to get wholesome nutrition while keeping calories, fat, and cholesterol low. When you break open an egg, you know it is fresh if the yolk holds its shape; as eggs age, the white thins and the yolk flattens.

Combat Meaty Cravings with Umami

Yes, you can "meat" your protein needs with plant foods, but people crave the *flavor* of meat. That meaty flavor has a name—*umami*. Umami (oo-MAH-mee) is the Japanese word for *savory* or *meaty*. It is considered the fifth taste (the first four are sweet, sour, salty, and bitter) and is common in meats and fish but is also present in some vegetables. When people cut meat out of their diets without replacing the umami taste, they can feel dissatisfied, as though something is missing. It's not the meat—it's the umami.

So as you cut back on meat, it is important to include vegetarian, umami-rich foods to get your fill of the meaty, savory flavor. You have eaten vegetarian, umami foods many times already: sautéed *mushrooms*, *tomato* sauce on pizza, or *Parmesan cheese* on pasta. I've asked my chef friends about this fifth taste element, and they get a sparkle in their eye and tell me it is one of the best-kept culinary secrets. See the Flex Box Craving Meaty Flavor? Add These Vegetarian Umami Foods for a list of all the vegetarian umami foods to add to your meals if you start craving meaty flavor.

Flex Fundamentals Group 1: Meet the New Meat Summary

- Vegetarian protein foods include legumes (e.g., beans, peas, lentils), nuts, and seeds.
- Each bean, pea, and lentil has a different and delicious taste and texture. I love legumes!
- You can fend off flatulence, gas, and toots if you take baby bean steps, chew, and try an enzyme helper.
- Don't say the *t* word (*tofu*). Call it "veggie white meat" to reduce the negative stigma attached to this versatile culinary chameleon.
- Veggie white meat (tofu) has a cousin named "tempeh," which is a soybean product with a very meaty texture.
- Go ahead and fake it—try veggie versions of burgers, ground meat, and sausages.
- Eat a healthy handful of nuts and seeds, not just for the crunch of it, but because they are full of heart-smart fat.
- Break an egg. They can be a healthy protein food for flexitarians, and you can prepare them in dozens and dozens of ways.
- If you crave the *flavor* of meat, add vegetarian foods that have umami (oo-MAH-mee), the Japanese word for "savory" or "meaty."
- This food group should be about 25 percent of your meals.

FLEX BOX

Craving Meaty Flavor? Add These Vegetarian Umami Foods

Aged cheese such as Parmesan
Beets
Broccoli
Cabbage
Carrots
Corn
Green peppers
Green tea
Mushrooms
Peas
Potatoes
Seaweed
Soy beans
Soy sauce
Spinach
Sweet potatoes
Tomatoes
Truffles
Walnuts

Flex Food Group 2: Veg Out and Satisfy Your Fruit Tooth

Everyone has heard that produce protects you from every chronic disease and is the most powerful group of foods on the planet. If we eat the recommended amount of fruits and veggies—at least 2 cups of fruit and 2½ cups of vegetables each day—we can live longer and have decreased risk of obesity, heart disease, cancer, diabetes, high blood pressure, heart attacks, and strokes. So if everyone knows that eating your fruits and veggies is healthy—how come only one out of ten eats the recommended daily dose of fruits and vegetables? The major perceived barriers to getting our reds, oranges, yellows, purples, and greens are taste, time, and cost. So in this section I am going to give you ideas for how to make your fruits and veggies more *tasty*, *quick*, and *cost controlled*. A good rule of thumb is that 50 percent of your grocery cart and 50 percent of your meals and snacks should come from this group.

I will also address the hot topic of organics and how to wash produce right to prevent *E. coli* and other bacteria from making you sick. At the end of this section, there is also a produce pop quiz to make sure you are getting enough variety in your fruits and veggies.

Three Tasty Tips to Make Vegetables Delicious

1. **Debitter with sugar, fat, and cooking.** Some people are very sensitive to bitter tastes and may be more prone to disliking the taste of naturally bitter vegetables. When preparing vegetables for yourself or someone who doesn't love the taste, aim to add moderate amounts of *sweet* condiments (e.g., barbecue sauce or sweet and sour sauce) or *fats* such as nuts or cheese (e.g., almonds in green beans or cheddar on broccoli) to make them more palate pleasing. Cooking vegetables also brings out natural sugars, so sauté, steam, microwave, bake, roast, or grill them to take the bitter edge off.
2. **Flavor-flavor training.** Research shows that when you pair a *liked* food flavor with an *unliked* food, over time you will start to authentically enjoy the unliked food flavor. Here's an example: if a child

Fact Stack

Cooking also makes fruit sweeter, so if you buy fruit that isn't quite ripe or sweet enough, cook it to release more natural sweetness. I spray or brush a little oil on cut fruit and then grill it (flesh side down) or broil it in the oven (flesh side up) for about six to eight minutes.

doesn't like spinach but loves ranch dressing, pizza, and pasta, try pairing spinach with any of those desired foods—in time, spinach will be a favorite flavor.

3. **Patience and persistence.** Even though you might not like a food the first time you eat it or the first way it is prepared, don't give up. Repeated exposure to a disliked food prepared in different ways is key to retraining adults' and children's minds and taste buds to like it. Research suggests that it can take up to fourteen times of eating a food before you begin to enjoy and prefer it. The moral of the story is have patience and persistence, because the food you once plugged your nose to eat will soon be what you crave!

Naturally Delicious Fruit Desserts

Put out a fruit bowl and not only do you have a pretty centerpiece, but you also will increase your fruit consumption. Anytime a food becomes easily accessible and available, you are more likely to eat it—in sight, in mouth! I also recommend keeping a hefty stash of bagged, unsweetened frozen fruit. Empty a bag of frozen fruit into a bowl or container, cover it, and stick it in the fridge. After it thaws, you can easily scoop some onto yogurt, oatmeal, or desserts. If you find your sweet tooth flares in the late afternoon, try to have 2 cups of fruit spread early in the day to suppress your sweet cravings *before* they occur.

Fresh or unsweetened frozen fruits are always the best choice because dried fruits and juices have more concentrated calories. I love dried fruit, so I have a rule that I follow—or at least try to most of the time: "Dried fruit for condiment use only." A tablespoon here and there on oatmeal, salads, and other dishes is not as calorie careless as eating the stuff straight from a bag.

Fresh fruit is a naturally sweet snack, but sometimes the fruit bowl just isn't enough to soothe your sugar cravings. So try my fancy fruit dessert recipes in Part Three to naturally tame that ferocious sweet tooth, such as Broiled Banana with Walnuts, Apple and Cranberry Skillet Crisp, Almond-Stuffed Dates, Cinnamon-Spice Peaches with Pecans, Dark-Chocolate-Dipped Apricots, Peach-Raspberry Crepes, and Pineapple with Candied Ginger and Pecans.

Convenience Increases Consumption

The easier it is to grab a food, the more likely you are to eat it. Make healthy fruits and veggies easy to grab, and it will make your job of eating healthier so much easier. Here are two ways to make your produce easy to grab:

1. **Precut and frozen.** Nothing saves time more than having someone else do your prep work. Buy precut and cleaned lettuce, carrots, grape tomatoes, cabbage, peapods, broccoli, cauliflower, and so on. Frozen produce is great, too, because it is already cut and cleaned. If you don't buy produce precut and ready to eat, chop it up yourself right when you get home from the store. Even though washed and cut produce doesn't last as long in the fridge, you will eat more if it is ready-to-go.
2. **Cook once, eat thrice.** This is a very useful tip. Anytime you make a salad or roast or grill vegetables—always make extra to have around for a couple of days. If you have a tray of leftover grilled vegetables in

> ***Feeling Good***
>
> Add twenty minutes of relaxation to your bedtime routine. Research has found that people can lose 2 pounds within the first eight days of adding relaxation before bed, because it can significantly reduce the number of nights you snack.

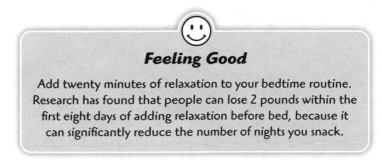

your fridge, you can toss them on a hummus sandwich, throw them into a pasta dish, or wrap them in a tortilla with beans.

Cost Control

To meet the fruit and vegetable guidelines, a family of four has to spend about $34.40 each week on produce. There are three ways to decrease produce costs:

1. **Buy produce at warehouse discount stores.** Shopping at bulk stores rather than independent or chain grocery stores can save almost $250 a year. If you are going to an independent or national store, be sure to shop from the sales paper and use their store discount cards if available.
2. **Shop in season for the best-tasting produce at the most reasonable prices.** See the Flex Box Seasonal Fruits and Vegetables (on page 38) for a general guide to seasonal produce.
3. **Reduce waste.** In my experience, the number one reason why fruits and vegetables are expensive is because of waste. Decreasing wasted produce is your ticket to saving money. You can decrease waste in two ways:

    - *Try the "fresh first, frozen follows" trick.* Purchase fresh and frozen produce—get enough *fresh* for only the first four to five days and then also get *frozen* for filling in the time between grocery store trips. Frozen produce is just as nutritious as fresh but can last up to twelve months in the freezer without going to waste. Just be sure to get the frozen vegetables *without* added salt, seasoning, or fat and fruits without added sugar.

Time Crunch

Keep an everyday veggie tray in your fridge. You don't have to wait for a party to enjoy a veggie tray. Keep easy-to-dip veggies such as grape tomatoes, baby carrots, cucumber slices, and peapods with a container of low-fat ranch dip at eye level in the fridge. Take the tray out for anytime easy munching.

- *Keep produce at eye level in your fridge, not in the crisper drawers or on lower shelves.* Crisper drawers take too much pulling and bending to open, and you can easily forget what's in there! If fruits and vegetables are right at eye level when you open the fridge, they will flash a subliminal message to you, saying, "Eat me, eat me."

The Big O? Organic Versus Conventional

The use of the term *organic* is regulated by the USDA. Organic food is grown without the use of conventional pesticides, fertilizers, synthetic hormones, or antibiotics; however, the USDA makes *no* claims that organic food is safer or more nutritious than conventional food. My opinion is that nine out of ten people don't eat enough produce, so the first step is to eat it, whether it is organic or not. Once you get your 2 cups of fruit and 2½ cups of vegetables every day, then you can consider purchasing all or some organic produce.

Wash Right—How to Ensure Your Produce Is Squeaky Clean

The USDA gives three steps for correctly handling produce to cut down on food-borne illness:

1. **Wash hands for twenty seconds with warm soapy water.** Proper hand washing can prevent many cases of food-borne illness.
2. **Wash produce with running water.** Under running water or your faucet spray nozzle, rub the produce with your hands or a scrub brush until the surface dirt (along with bacteria) is removed. Running water has an abrasive effect that soaking doesn't. Use the scrub brush for the firm produce such as cucumbers, melons, and carrots. Wash even the produce you are going to peel, such as avocados, kiwi, and squash because the peel can contaminate the parts you are going to eat. Note: it is not recommended that you use soap, detergent, or commercial washes.
3. **Wipe produce with a clean paper towel to further reduce bacteria.** This step wipes off additional bacteria that may be on produce even after it has been scrubbed under water.

FLEX BOX

Seasonal Fruits and Vegetables

Year Round

Avocados
Bananas
Bell peppers
Cabbage
Carrots
Celery
Lemons
Lettuce
Onions
Papayas
Potatoes

Spring

Apricots
Artichokes
Asparagus
Broccoli
Chives
Collard greens
English peas
Fava beans
Fennel
Fiddlehead ferns
Green beans
Honeydew
Limes
Mango
Morel mushrooms
Mustard greens
Oranges
Peapods
Pineapple
Ramps
Rhubarb
Snow peas
Sorrel
Spinach
Spring baby lettuce
Strawberries
Sugar snap peas
Sweet corn
Swiss chard
Vidalia onions
Watercress

Summer

Apricots
Beets
Bell peppers
Blackberries
Blueberries
Boysenberries
Cantaloupe
Casaba melon
Cherries
Crenshaw melon
Cucumbers
Eggplant
Figs
Garlic
Grapefruit
Grapes
Green beans
Green peas
Honeydew melon
Kiwi
Lima beans
Limes
Loganberries
Nectarines
Okra
Peaches
Persian melons
Plums
Radishes
Raspberries
Strawberries
Summer squash
Sweet corn
Tomatillos
Tomatoes
Watermelon
Zucchini

Fall

Acorn squash	Cranberries	Persimmons
Apples	Daikon radish	Pineapple
Belgian endive	Garlic	Pomegranate
Bok choy	Ginger	Pumpkin
Broccoli	Grapes	Quince
Brussels sprouts	Guava	Rutabagas
Butternut squash	Huckleberries	Sweet potatoes
Cauliflower	Kohlrabi	Swiss chard
Celery root	Kumquats	Turnips
Chayote squash	Mushrooms	Winter squash
Cherimoya	Parsnips	Yams
Coconuts	Pear	

Winter

Apples	Kale	Red currants
Belgian endive	Leeks	Rutabagas
Bok choy	Mushrooms	Sweet potatoes
Brussels sprouts	Oranges	Tangerines
Cherimoya	Parsnips	Turnips
Chestnuts	Pear	Winter squash
Coconut	Persimmons	Yams
Dates	Pummelo	
Grapefruit	Radicchio	

Adapted from the Centers for Disease Control and fruitsandveggiesmorematters.org.

Feeling Good

Fantasize about healthy food. Imagine eating a cold, crisp, and juicy apple and enjoying it. Remind yourself how good you feel after healthy homemade vegetable burritos instead of greasy takeout. When your make yourself think eating healthy food is delicious (even if you don't completely believe it), it is easier to make healthy food decisions.

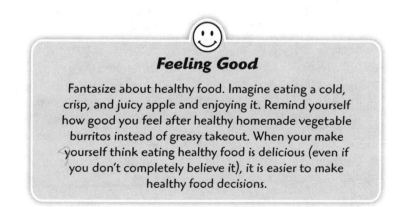

Produce Pop Quiz: Do You Eat Enough Variety?

Dietary variety is associated with a more nutritious diet. Test your fruit and vegetable variety. Put a check mark by each fruit and vegetable you have eaten over the past month:

Fruits

- ☐ Apple
- ☐ Apricot
- ☐ Avocado
- ☐ Banana
- ☐ Blackberry
- ☐ Blueberry
- ☐ Cantaloupe
- ☐ Cherry
- ☐ Cranberry
- ☐ Currant
- ☐ Date
- ☐ Fig
- ☐ Grape
- ☐ Grapefruit
- ☐ Guava
- ☐ Honeydew
- ☐ Kiwi
- ☐ Kumquat
- ☐ Mango
- ☐ Nectarine
- ☐ Orange
- ☐ Papaya
- ☐ Passion fruit
- ☐ Peach
- ☐ Pear
- ☐ Persimmon
- ☐ Pineapple
- ☐ Plum
- ☐ Pomegranate
- ☐ Quince
- ☐ Raspberry
- ☐ Strawberry
- ☐ Tangerine
- ☐ Watermelon

Vegetables

- ☐ Artichoke
- ☐ Arugula
- ☐ Asparagus
- ☐ Bean (legumes)
- ☐ Beet
- ☐ Bok choy
- ☐ Broccoli
- ☐ Brussels sprout
- ☐ Cabbage
- ☐ Carrot
- ☐ Cauliflower
- ☐ Celery
- ☐ Corn
- ☐ Cucumber
- ☐ Eggplant
- ☐ Endive
- ☐ Fennel
- ☐ Fiddlehead fern
- ☐ Green bean
- ☐ Greens (collard, mustard, beet, dandelion, kale, Swiss chard)
- ☐ Jicama
- ☐ Kohlrabi
- ☐ Leek
- ☐ Lettuce

Vegetables (continued)

- ☐ Mushroom
- ☐ Okra
- ☐ Onion
- ☐ Parsnip
- ☐ Pea
- ☐ Pepper (sweet or spicy)
- ☐ Radicchio
- ☐ Radish
- ☐ Ramp
- ☐ Rhubarb
- ☐ Rutabaga
- ☐ Salsify
- ☐ Shallot
- ☐ Spinach
- ☐ Sprouts (alfalfa, mung bean, clover, BroccoSprouts)
- ☐ Summer squash
- ☐ Sunchoke
- ☐ Sweet potato
- ☐ Tomatillo
- ☐ Tomato
- ☐ Turnip
- ☐ Watercress
- ☐ White potato
- ☐ Winter squash (pumpkin, acorn, butternut, spaghetti)
- ☐ Zucchini

Now look over your list. To start adding in more variety, aim to buy at least one of the fruits and vegetables you did not check off. If you don't know what to do with one of the more unusual produce items and it is not in this book, visit websites such as fruitsandveggiesmorematters.org, or books such as *Field Guide to Produce*, by Aliza Green, or *Encyclopedia of Foods*, published by Academic Press, for pictures and suggestions.

Flex Fundamentals Group 2: Veg Out and Satisfy Your Fruit Tooth Summary

- Use three tasty tricks to get your vegetables to taste better: (1) debitter with sugar, fat, and cooking, (2) try flavor-flavor training, and (3) practice patience and persistence.
- Enjoy naturally delicious fruit-based desserts.
- Control costs by going to warehouse stores, shopping seasonally, and reducing waste with the "fresh first, frozen follows" trick and easy eye-level storage.
- Keep produce convenient by using precut and frozen versions and the "cook once, eat thrice" tip.
- Nine out of ten people don't eat enough produce every day, so worry about eating enough first and then worry about the big "O" (organic).

- Clean your produce with a running-water rub, followed by a paper towel wipe down.
- Take the produce pop quiz to make sure you are getting enough variety.
- This group should make up at least 50 percent of your meals and snacks.

Fact Stack

Vary your veggies. We need at least 2½ cups of vegetables each day, and over the course of the week, our veggie variety should look like this:

Dark green vegetables: 3 cups per week (e.g., broccoli, spinach, romaine lettuce, collard and mustard greens, kale, etc.)

Orange vegetables: 2 cups per week (e.g., carrots, sweet potatoes, winter squash, pumpkins, etc.)

Legumes: 3 cups per week (e.g., pinto beans, kidney beans, lentils, chickpeas, tofu, etc.)

Starchy vegetables: 3 cups per week (e.g., white potatoes, corn, peas, etc.)

Other vegetables: 6½ cups per week (e.g., tomatoes, green beans, onions, mushrooms, etc.).

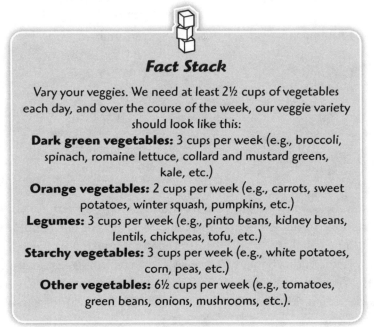

Flex Food Group 3: Go with the Grain

Whole grains are an important source of many nutrients, such as fiber, B vitamins (thiamine, riboflavin, niacin, and folate), and minerals (iron, magnesium, and selenium). Including whole grains as part of a healthy diet reduces the risk of heart disease and some types of cancer, and corrects constipation. It is estimated that eating whole grains regularly reduces risk of stroke, type 2 diabetes, and heart disease by almost 30 percent. People who eat whole grains tend to weigh less than people who don't eat them.

A whole grain has three parts: bran, germ, and endosperm. Refined or processed grains have the bran and germ removed, so they have less fiber, vitamins, minerals, antioxidants, and healthy fats. If you choose processed grains, you will miss out on 25 percent of the grain's protein and about fifteen key nutrients found in the bran and germ. There is only *one* way to be sure you are purchasing a whole grain—look at the *ingredient list* and buy products that have the word *whole*. When you see the word *enriched* on a package, that means the grain has been processed and vitamins and minerals were added back—this is *not* a whole-grain product. Buy whole-grain versions of your favorite foods, such as pasta, cereal, crackers, pitas, pancake mixes, tortillas, rolls, and bread.

You can prepare a whole world of uncommon whole grains by boiling and simmering them in water until they are tender with a delicate chewiness. Out-of-the-ordinary whole grains such as barley, millet, quinoa, and bulgur are delicious, and cooking them is just like cooking more common whole grains such as oatmeal and brown rice. Each grain takes a different amount of water and time to cook. See the Flex Box Whole-Grain Cooking Guide for whole-grain cooking basics. Trying different whole grains helps keep your food interesting (boring food can sabotage your healthy eating efforts!), and since each grain has a slightly different nutrient profile, the variety helps you achieve optimum nutrition.

In the section to follow I will review some of the whole grains that I use regularly, which include barley, corn, millet, oat, quinoa, rice,

FLEX BOX

Whole-Grain Cooking Guide

Bring 1 cup uncooked grains and recommended amount of water to a boil. Cover pot and simmer for recommended time. If you are cooking less than 1 cup of grain, it will take slightly less time; if cooking more than 1 cup, it will take a little longer.

Grain (1 cup, uncooked)	**Water** (in cups)	**Simmer Time** (in minutes)	**Yield** (in cups)
Amaranth	2	25	3½
Barley, hulled	3	45–60	3½
Buckwheat (kasha)	2	20	4
Bulgur (cracked wheat)	2	15	2½
Cornmeal (polenta)	4	30	2½
Kamut (presoak*)	4	45–60	3
Millet	2½	30	4
Oats, rolled	2	5	2½
Oats, steel cut	3	30	3
Oats, whole groats (presoak*)	4	60	3
Quinoa	2	15	3½
Rice, brown	2½	40	3½
Rye (presoak*)	4	45–60	3
Sorghum	4	40	3
Spelt (presoak*)	4	45–60	3
Teff	4	20	3
Triticale (presoak*)	3	45	3
Wheat, berries (presoak*)	4	45–60	3
Wheat, whole wheat couscous	1½	15	3
Wild rice	3	50	3½

Note: If your grains are too watery or soggy (mine often are because I tend not to measure the water—I just fill up the pot with 1 cup of grain and lots of water), just strain them to remove the excess water.

**Presoak* means to cover grains with water in a pot and keep them covered in the fridge for 6 to 8 hours or overnight before cooking. Change water, and then cook according to the preceding chart.

Adapted from the Whole Grain Council (wholegrainscouncil.org).

wheat, and a variety of whole-grain products such as pasta, pitas, waffles, wraps, and bread. A good rule of thumb is that 25 percent of your grocery cart and 25 percent of your meals should come from this group.

Once you start cooking with a variety of whole grains, I encourage you to go beyond the grains I detail in this book and explore grains such as amaranth, buckwheat, kamut, rye, spelt, sorghum, teff, and triticale. You can find these whole grains in some conventional grocery stores, in health food stores, or online at bobsredmill.com (Bob's Red Mill is a great resource for finding whole grains and recipes) or amazon.com.

Note: it is estimated that 1 in 133 Americans have a condition known as celiac disease. People with celiac disease have to avoid gluten (a protein in certain grains) because it sets off an abnormal autoimmune response, which damages the small intestines and leads to nutrient deficiencies. See the Flex Box Grains with Gluten Guide for a list of grains that contain gluten.

Barley

You will find two kinds of barley at the store, hulled and pearled. Buy *hulled* because it is whole grain; the pearled version has the bran removed. Whole barley is not the quickest grain—it takes a while to cook (forty-five to sixty minutes)—but the texture and taste are well worth the time

FLEX BOX

Grains with Gluten Guide

Barley
Kamut
Rye
Spelt
Triticale
Wheat (products such as bulgur, couscous, and durum pasta flour)

Note: Oats are a tricky one—some sources say oats should be avoided, while others say oats are fine. If you are on a gluten-free diet, consider purchasing oats that are processed and labeled "gluten-free."

investment. Barley has the U.S. Food and Drug Administration's (FDA) stamp of approval as a heart-healthy food. It contains a heart-healthy compound called beta-glucan, which significantly lowers bad, LDL (low-density lipoprotein) cholesterol. A great tip is to make a large batch of barley once and refrigerate it for up to five days or freeze cooked barley leftovers in 1-cup containers for three to six months. Another clever idea is to use your slow cooker—put barley (or any longer-cooking grain) and water on low while you sleep or are at work.

Corn

There are three major types or varieties of corn grown in the United States: sweet corn, field corn, and popcorn. Sweet corn is eaten as a vegetable, popcorn is eaten as a popular snack food, and field corn is made into hominy (posole), grits, masa, masa harina, cornmeal, and polenta. To make sure your corn products are whole grain, look for the word *whole* in the ingredient list. If you see the word *degerminated* (germ removed), it is not whole grain. If you see the words *limed corn* (or *lye*) on the ingredient list, that means the corn has been processed and is not whole grain. Limed corn is not whole grain, but it does have more niacin (B vitamin) and calcium than unprocessed versions, so you don't necessarily have to snub it. Here's a quick explanation of various corn products:

- *Hominy* (also known as posole) is corn that has undergone the lime process and is not a whole grain.
- *Grits* are not usually whole grain.
- Freshly cooked hominy can be made into a dough called *masa*. Masa can be dried and ground into flour called *masa harina*. Both masa and masa harina are commonly used to make tamales, tortillas, and corn chips (not usually whole grain).
- *Polenta* is made from *cornmeal* and is not necessarily whole grain. Check the ingredients to make sure it says "whole" cornmeal.

Millet

Millet is a tiny, delicate grain that easily takes on the flavor of what it is cooked with. It can have two distinct textures: if millet is just left alone

Fact Stack

Get seven to eight hours of sleep. Not getting enough sleep is associated with hormonal changes such as decreased leptin levels and increased ghrelin, which may increase appetite. Women who sleep five hours or less are 32 percent more likely to gain weight than those who get seven to eight hours of nightly z's.

and not stirred during simmering, the grains will be separate like rice, but if you stir it while it is cooking, it will become creamy—almost like mashed potatoes.

Oats

I have to admit I am an oatmeal pusher. Oatmeal is a classic heart-smart food with more than forty years of research confirming that it lowers cholesterol. Oatmeal has been shown to be one of the most filling breakfasts. Its fabulous filling potential is a result of cooking water into the grain—anytime you cook water into a food (think of soups and other whole grains such as barley and rice), it is more filling than a dry food (such as toast, cold cereal, or a bagel).

I prefer the texture of old-fashioned (rolled) oats or steel-cut oats, but you don't have to worry if you only have time for instant oatmeal packets; even those are whole grain. See the Flex Box Oat Overview for an oat explanation. If you decide to use the longer-cooking types, you can make a large batch once and refrigerate it for up to five days or freeze cooked oatmeal leftovers in 1-cup containers for three to six months. Another clever idea is to use your slow cooker—put oat groats, steel-cut oats, or old-fashioned (rolled) oats plus water (use 1 to 2 extra cups of water than usual so it doesn't dry out) on low while you sleep, and wake up to a hot breakfast.

The granola you buy in the store often is made with rolled oats but is high in calories because of added fat and sugar. A healthier option is *muesli* (German for "mixture"), which is a blend of raw oats, fruit, and nuts usually without added fat and sugar. Do-it-yourself (DIY)

FLEX BOX

Oat Overview

All versions are *whole* grain:

Oat groats: whole oat kernels (longest cooking)
Steel-cut or Irish: oat groats cut into smaller pieces
Old-fashioned or rolled: oat groats steamed and pressed flat
Quick-cooking: oat groats cut into smaller pieces before being steamed and pressed flat
Instant: oats precooked, dried, and pressed thin (fastest cooking)

---

muesli is made by mixing a half cup of raw (*uncooked*) rolled oats with a couple tablespoons of your favorite dried fruit, nuts, or both. I prefer my muesli soft and tender, so I let it soak in an equal part of milk, soy milk, kefir, or yogurt for ten minutes or overnight in the fridge—no cooking necessary! Soaking your muesli in the fridge is a great option for those warm-weather days when you don't feel like eating a bowl of hot oatmeal.

Quinoa

Quinoa is pronounced "keen-wa" and nutritionally can be considered a supergrain because it has more iron than other grains and is a good source of potassium, riboflavin, magnesium, folate, and zinc. It is also high in protein: 1 cup cooked has 6 to 7 grams of protein (as much as one egg). Quinoa is one of the fastest-cooking and most versatile grains. I call quinoa the "gateway grain" because once people try it, they want to experiment with more types of whole grains.

Rice

Brown rice is a very popular whole grain found in every grocery store. Rice is classified primarily by the size of the grain. Brown *long*-grain rice is long, is slender, and becomes fluffy and separate; *medium*-grain is shorter, is plumper, and is a good all-purpose rice; and *short* grain is almost round and very sticky. There are also specialty varieties of rice such as basmati and jasmine (choose these in brown-rice versions). If you don't have much time, companies such as Trader Joe's, Birds Eye, and Uncle Ben's have sixty- to ninety-*second* microwavable brown rice. These are good in a pinch, but the texture is not quite as good as simmering your own for forty minutes. *Wild rice* technically is neither rice nor a grain but rather a grass seed. Nutritionally, it has about double the protein of other rice and more B vitamins and zinc.

Mochi (MO-chee) is made from sticky brown rice that is steamed, mashed, and pressed into flat sheets. A company named Grainaissance (grainaissance.com) makes various flavors of mochi such as pizza, chocolate brownie, and raisin cinnamon. Mochi can be found in the refrigerated section of many health food stores. After it is cut and baked, it puffs up and can be eaten as is or stuffed with your favorite ingredients.

Wheat

Wheat is a very common whole grain. Many products are available in whole wheat versions, such as pasta, pitas, waffles, bread, buns, English muffins, bagels, and wraps. If you are a Cream of Wheat (farina) lover, unfortunately it is not whole grain. But the good news is that this book has plenty of hot, *whole*-grain breakfast recipes you can try instead!

The most whole form of wheat is called wheat berries. They are delicious but have to be soaked overnight and then simmered for forty-five minutes. They have a great nutty, chewy texture. If you want to use wheat

Fact Stack

Turn off the tube. Tube addicts who watch more than two hours of daily TV eat 137 more calories per day than those who watch less.

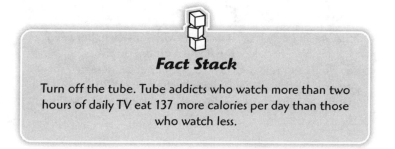

berries, you can take a recipe from this book and just swap the grain. For example, the Curried Quinoa Salad recipe (see Index) can easily become a Curried Wheat Berry Salad! When wheat berries are cracked into smaller pieces, they are called *bulgur* (cracked wheat). Bulgur has the same nutrition and nutty taste (but not the same firm, hardy texture) as wheat berries, but it takes only fifteen minutes to cook.

Pasta

Most pasta is made from wheat, although you can find pasta made from other grains and blends such as rice, corn, quinoa, spelt, or buckwheat. In fact, my husband is very proud he found us pasta made with eight 100 percent whole grains (Racconto brand): wheat, rye, buckwheat, Kamut, spelt, millet, barley, and brown rice. Make sure you get the whole-grain version of pasta, by checking the ingredients to see the word *whole*, such as in "whole durum wheat." Pasta is a great way to enjoy whole grains because it cooks quickly and comes in so many shapes, such as couscous (yes, this is minipasta!), orzo (this looks like rice), penne, rigatoni, fettuccine, and the list goes on and on.

A good rule of thumb is to have about 1 cup of cooked pasta (around 200 calories) at a meal and then add beans or another lean protein and plenty of veggies to make the meal more filling. I've included plenty of flexitarian pasta recipes because they are always a favorite—they are the most requested recipes from the magazine editors I work with and from my cooking-class participants.

Fact Stack

Eat meals every four to six hours with a snack in between. Eating on schedule is the single most important thing you can do to control your cravings and appetite. Research shows people who have a regular eating schedule eat 80 calories less per day than those who skip meals and eat at irregular times.

Bread and Beyond

You can purchase waffles, flatbreads, pitas, bread, and wraps made from whole grains. Often these products are made with whole wheat, but sometimes they are made with a blend of whole grains such as brown rice, whole oats, whole barley, whole triticale, whole rye, whole buckwheat, whole millet, and so on. If you don't anticipate using the entire package in a week's time, you can freeze these products for three to six months; wrap them tightly to prevent freezer burn. Just move the amount you need for the week to the fridge so it can thaw and be ready to use. To pick the best brands of these products, follow this three-step process:

1. Check ingredients: look for the word *whole* to make sure you are getting the real deal.
2. Check calories: compare similar whole-grain brands and choose the lower-calorie items.
3. Check fiber: aim for 3 to 5 grams per serving or more.

Exploring Other Grains

I have highlighted some of the whole grains I use regularly (e.g., barley, corn, millet, oat, quinoa, rice, and wheat), but there is a whole world of whole grains you can explore. Many of the following grains are longer cooking and may require soaking overnight before cooking. Check the Flex Box Whole-Grain Cooking Guide for cooking directions.

- **Amaranth** (AM-ah-ranth): a tiny grain about the size of a poppy seed. It cooks into a thick, super-sticky texture, which can be good for breakfast porridge or even added to soups as a thickener. You can also put raw amaranth into recipes such as cookies and muffins for an unexpected crunch.
- **Buckwheat:** the whole, unprocessed form is called buckwheat groats. When the groats are roasted and sometimes cracked, they are called kasha. For an easy way to try buckwheat, buy 100 percent buckwheat noodles (soba noodles) to serve alongside stir-fried veggies.

- **Kamut** (kah-MOOT): an early variety of wheat with larger kernels and a rich, buttery flavor. It has more protein, magnesium, and zinc than whole wheat.
- **Rye:** a familiar ingredient in rye bread (although most rye bread is primarily wheat flour with just a bit of rye). Unprocessed rye berries have a hearty taste that goes well blended with other grains such as brown rice or hulled barley. Mixing various cooked grains together (called grain medleys) is a hot culinary trend!
- **Sorghum:** also known as milo. It can be bought as whole, unprocessed sorghum berries (which look a bit like millet) or as a flour with a delicate, almost sweet taste.
- **Spelt:** an early variety of wheat with a light and nutty flavor. It is higher in protein than whole wheat.
- **Teff:** a very tiny grain that is a staple in Ethiopia. Its texture is slightly sticky and a little crunchy, and it has a light, sweet, and nutty taste.
- **Triticale** (trih-tih-KAY-lee): a hybrid mix of wheat and rye. You may have already eaten triticale in products from companies such as Kashi and Arrowhead Mills, because they use it in their whole-grain blends.
- **Wheat berries:** also called wheat groats, although I think calling them wheat berries is more pleasant. They are whole, unprocessed wheat kernels. Although already mentioned in the wheat section, this favorite of mine is worth mentioning again here.

Flex Fundamentals Group 3: Go with the Grain Summary

- Whole grains have three wholesome parts: bran, germ, and endosperm.
- There is only *one* way to ensure you are buying whole grains; read the ingredients for the word *whole*.
- Enjoy tried-and-true favorites: barley, corn, millet, oat, quinoa, rice, and wheat.
- Explore and experiment with other whole grains (even if you can't pronounce them): amaranth, buckwheat, Kamut, rye, sorghum, spelt, teff, and triticale.
- This food group should be about 25 percent of your meals.

Flex Food Group 4: Dairy Discovery

Think dairy, and three main foods come to mind: milk, cheese, and yogurt. We typically think of these products as made from cow's milk, but they can come from other animals (e.g., sheep and goat) and can be made from plant foods such as nuts, rice, and soy. Aim to have two to three servings (about 8 ounces each) of dairy per day. This section is an overview of your milk, cheese, and yogurt options.

Milk

Cows' milk is a nutrient-rich food providing calcium, vitamin D, protein, potassium, vitamin A, vitamin B_{12}, riboflavin, niacin, and phosphorus. Studies have linked adequate dairy foods such as milk with bone and dental health and decreased risk of obesity, hypertension, diabetes, heart disease, stroke, and colon and breast cancers. If you opt out of the animal-based milk, be sure to include *enriched* versions of soy, rice, and almond milk in your daily routine. *Enriched* means that the milk has important added nutrients: calcium, vitamin D, vitamin B_{12}, vitamin A, and sometimes the B vitamin riboflavin. Choose enriched plant-based milk that meets three criteria per cup: (1) 70 to 80 calories, (2) 6 to 7 grams of protein, and (3) 30 percent calcium plus 25 percent vitamin D. Including animal or enriched plant-based milk is an easy way to get key nutrients into your diet, so keep your fridge stocked with it weekly.

Fact Stack

You are only as healthy as your last trip to the grocery store. Shop once a week to keep your home stocked with healthy foods. Your grocery cart should have 50 percent produce, 25 percent whole grains, and 25 percent lean proteins and low-fat dairy foods.

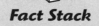

Cheese

Cheese is a *fresh* or *ripened* (aged) product made from coagulated milk. *Fresh* cheeses such as cottage, ricotta, cream, and farmer (drained and pressed cottage cheese) have higher moisture content and tend to be lower in fat and sodium than other cheeses. There are countless *ripened* cheeses categorized by textures such as hard (Parmesan), semifirm (cheddar), semisoft (Gouda), soft-ripened (Brie), and blue-veined (Gorgonzola). Cheese can be made from the milk of animals such as cows, sheep, or goats and also can be made from plants such as almonds, rice, or soy. Cheese is usually high in protein and contains calcium.

Even within one variety of cheese, variations in the type of milk, processing, season, and locality can lead to marked fluctuations in nutrition composition. Generally, cheese can be fairly high in sodium and saturated fat (the artery-clogging type), so when choosing cheese, opt for brands with *saturated* fat levels of about 4 grams or less per serving. In my practice I have seen many vegetarians who are cheeseaholics. Cheese is delicious and adds flavor, but it also adds sodium and fat. So use it sparingly—only an ounce a day and not every day. Choose flavorful cheeses so a little can go a long way toward enhancing your food.

A fantastic cheese substitute is *yogurt cheese.* You can make yogurt cheese by lining a colander with several folds of cheesecloth, paper towels, a kitchen towel, or coffee filters. Pour plain, low-fat yogurt into the lined colander, cover it, and let it drain into a bowl overnight in the refrigerator—you get a thick, creamy, cheeselike product. Add chopped herbs for a fresh and savory cracker spread, or make it a sweet fruit dip with spices, honey, or maple syrup.

Note: pregnant women are discouraged from eating unpasteurized soft cheeses such as feta, goat, Brie, Camembert, blue-veined cheese (e.g., Gorgonzola, blue), and Mexican *queso fresco* because of the potential for these cheeses to hold bacteria called *listeria.*

Yogurt

Yogurt not only has the nutritional benefits of milk, but it also has billions of healthy bacteria called probiotics. You can think of probiotics as soldiers ready to fight lactose intolerance, diarrhea, constipation and infections and even help boost your immune system. Look on yogurt containers for the National Yogurt Association's "Live and Active Cultures" seal, which means there are at least two types of healthy bacteria and 100 million bacteria per gram at the time of manufacture.

Most yogurts are made from cow's milk, although soy yogurt is made from soy milk. Greek-style yogurt (usually made with cow's milk but also made from sheep's or goat's milk) is richer, creamier, and thicker than the standard version because it is strained to remove much of the liquid whey. The straining process concentrates the protein, so Greek-style yogurt has about 15 grams of protein per 6 ounces—double the protein of standard yogurt. Greek yogurt tends to have 100 to 200 milligrams less calcium per container than standard yogurt, but it is so low in calories and delicious that this isn't a deal breaker.

Buy plain, unsweetened, low-fat versions of yogurt. It isn't boring; it is a blank canvas in which you can add your own fruits for flavor and control your own sweetness level. One teaspoon of honey in 6 ounces of plain, low-fat yogurt is my favorite because it not only tastes delicious, but the honey feeds the good bacteria to make them even stronger and more beneficial.

Kefir. A close cousin of yogurt is kefir. Kefir (pronounced keh-FEER or KEY-fir) is fermented milk and is Turkish for "good feeling." It tastes like a thick, tangy milk shake and is perfect for smoothies. I also like kefir instead of milk for cereal or morning muesli. As with yogurt, buy plain, low-fat kefir.

Flex Fundamentals Group 4: Dairy Discovery Summary

- Dairy foods can come from animals such as cows or from plant foods such as soybeans.
- Flexitarians live in a world where animal-based and plant-based dairy foods can get along peacefully.
- Dairy foods such as yogurt and kefir contain bacteria that may have health benefits, such as enhancing the immune system to fight diseases.
- Higher-fat dairy foods, such as cheese, should be limited to an ounce or less per day.
- Aim to include animal- or plant-based dairy foods such as milk, cheese, yogurt, and kefir two to three times a day.

Flex Food Group 5: Sugar and Spice (and Everything in Between)

The bottom line is condiments make or break a healthy eating plan. With the right ones, healthy food sings with good nutrition and good taste. But the wrong condiments can drown your food in excess salt, sugar, and calories. Avoiding condiments can cause you to choke on dull, bland, blah food. In my professional opinion, condiments are so important I gave them their own food group! Take this food group seriously, and you will enjoy your Flex foods so much more.

The Baker's Dozen (Thirteen) Best for Your Spice Rack

It is important to have a well-stocked dry herb and spice rack to make your food taste great without adding calories or fat. Herbs are the leaves of plants, and spices are from the aromatic parts such as roots, bark, pods, fruits, seeds, berries, or flowers. Recent research shows herbs and spices are shockingly high in healthy antioxidants. So you get not only flavor from each dash and sprinkle but also amazing disease prevention. Dried herbs and ground spices start losing strength after about twelve months, so if it has been a while since you replaced them—go to the store! You can get the best deals and find the most variety of herbs and spices at specialty spice stores, not at your local grocer. Spice stores are very fun to browse and sniff around, but most

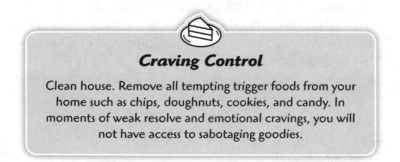

> ***Craving Control***
>
> Clean house. Remove all tempting trigger foods from your home such as chips, doughnuts, cookies, and candy. In moments of weak resolve and emotional cravings, you will not have access to sabotaging goodies.

of the time I have my spices and herbs delivered to my door from stores such as penzeys.com or thespicehouse.com.

Store spices in a cool, dark place. Humidity (by the dishwasher or in the fridge), light (out in the open), and heat (near the stove) cause herbs and spices to lose their flavor more quickly. I store mine in a drawer away from the dishwasher and stove. Herbs and spices also make great gifts—I've given them to everyone on my gift list. Here is my list of the baker's dozen (thirteen) must-haves, and I hope you experiment beyond these over time:

- **Buttermilk ranch seasoning:** herb blend of salt, bell peppers, garlic, onion, sugar, black pepper, parsley, thyme, and basil. You probably have to go to a spice specialty store (such as penzeys.com or thespicehouse.com) for this, but it is worth the trouble. You can season *any* type of vegetable with it and make delicious ranch dressings by stirring some in plain yogurt or low-fat sour cream. It doesn't contain monosodium glutamate (MSG), which is found in most of the dried ranch dressing packets you find in the grocery store.
- **Chili powder:** spice blend of chili peppers, cumin, garlic, and oregano. Of course, this tastes great in chili, but it's also great in most Mexican-type dishes like beans and rice and burritos.
- **Cinnamon:** spice. Cinnamon adds a natural sweet taste to foods. Cinnamon may decrease total cholesterol and glucose (blood sugar).
- **Crushed red chili pepper flakes:** spice. Hot peppers contain a chemical called capsaicin, which may decrease inflammation and pain, making this spice especially helpful in conditions such as arthritis. A spicy meal may slightly increase your metabolism to help you burn about 15 extra calories.
- **Cumin:** spice. You can buy ground or whole cumin seeds. I primarily use ground. It gives a warm and slightly earthy flavor to food.
- **Curry powder:** spice blend of turmeric, cumin, black pepper, ginger, coriander, garlic, cloves, and cayenne. All the spices in this blend are healthy, especially turmeric. Turmeric contains a chemical called curcumin, which may help prevent certain types of cancer (especially colon and skin), heart disease, and arthritis.

- **Italian seasoning:** herb blend of oregano, basil, thyme, rosemary, and marjoram. All the herbs in this blend are healthy, especially oregano. Oregano has more cancer-fighting antioxidants than almost all other herbs and spices.
- **Old Bay:** spice blend of celery salt, mustard, red pepper, black pepper, bay leaves, cloves, allspice, ginger, mace, cardamom, cinnamon, and paprika. This is not just for seafood; use it on vegetables for a little kick.
- **Smoky paprika:** spice. I used to think paprika was just a tasteless red powder to sprinkle on deviled eggs, but I have since come to find out that there are many types and flavors of paprika. Paprika has flavors from sweet to hot to smoky, depending on the type of pepper and processing.
- **Pie spice (apple or pumpkin):** spice blend of cinnamon, allspice, clove, ginger, and nutmeg. It is a great spice to add to foods for people who want to cut back on sugar but still want a mild sweet taste. All of the spices in this blend tend to fake your tongue into thinking you are eating sugar. Vanilla flavor also works for that sweet taste without sugar.
- **Salt and black pepper:** spices. These are the classics. Use salt sparingly, since one teaspoon has almost 2,400 milligrams sodium, the max we are supposed to have in a whole day. A pinch of salt (1⁄16 of a teaspoon) has 150 milligrams of sodium and brightens the flavor of food, so don't be afraid to do a dash. Sea salt is more mineral-rich than table salt and tends to have a less metallic taste because it isn't iodized. Sea salt has about the same amount of sodium as table salt; coarse-ground sea salt may have a little less per teaspoon because less fits on the measuring spoon. Black pepper is used in almost all cuisines of the world because it is a warm and slightly spicy addition to any dish. Grind your own whole black peppercorns if you want the most flavor.
- **Rosemary:** herb. This may help increase memory, and it tastes great on anything potato or tomato based!
- **Sage:** herb. The bottom line here is that sage makes foods taste like savory stuffing—not to mention that it is in the top two of high-antioxidant herbs and spices (oregano is the only herb that surpasses the disease-fighting antioxidant level of sage).

Feeling Good

Do something pleasurable every day. To help take your mind off of daily responsibility and to unwind, find nonfood joyful pleasures instead of emotional eating. Read popular magazines or a "trashy" novel, take a long shower, dance to your favorite song, or lounge on your bed with comfy slippers for at least fifteen minutes daily.

Magic Eight Fresh Herbs and Spices

Fresh herbs need a little tender loving care concerning storage, but they can last up to a week in the fridge if stored properly. Excess wetness can make them spoil faster, so keep them wrapped (like a burrito) in a dish towel or paper towel to absorb extra moisture. You don't have to buy each of these every week, but I would have at least two or three on hand. If you have too many fresh herbs, you can experiment with freezing them in ice cube trays: chop the fresh herbs into tiny pieces, fill an ice cube tray half-full with herbs, cover with cold water, and freeze. The herb cubes can be dropped directly into soups and sauces or defrosted and used in dressings and marinades.

- **Basil:** herb. Basil does more than give food fresh Italian flavor: it is rich in antioxidants to protect against chronic disease and is also an excellent source of vitamin K, which contributes to healthy blood and bones.
- **Chives:** herb. Chives are a delicate-flavored member of the onion family. Like onions they contain sulfur compounds that may prevent cancer. Store fresh chives for about three to four days in the warmest part of the fridge because they tend to freeze and rot easily. Don't bother with dried chives, as they have very little flavor.
- **Cilantro:** herb. Love it or hate it. Some dislike cilantro, because they claim it tastes like soap. For others, cilantro tastes lively and brightens up a meal. Note: *cilantro* refers to the fresh leaves, and *coriander* is the seed of the same plant.

- **Dill:** herb. Say "dill," and the word *pickle* comes to mind. Although I do enjoy pickles (classic cucumbers, carrots, cauliflower, and asparagus), dill's mildly sweet flavor can be paired with many other foods, such as fish, beans, yogurt, eggs, and beets, to name a few.
- **Garlic:** spice. The strong flavor of garlic may not help you in the friend department, but it will help you have a healthy heart. One of garlic's active ingredients, called allicin, has been shown to decrease cholesterol and lower blood pressure. Crush or chop garlic well before using it because it releases and activates the healthy ingredients, but garlic loses its power when overcooked. Just cook lightly, or use raw garlic. Aim to have one to two cloves of garlic each day for optimal health benefits.
- **Ginger:** spice. Ginger potentially relieves motion sickness and decreases nausea (especially during pregnancy). I think it is the perfect ingredient to include in desserts or after-dinner tea to settle your stomach.
- **Mint:** herb. Fresh breath is not all you can expect from adding mint to your recipes. Mint's naturally occurring active ingredients (called menthol and menthone) have calming effects on the intestinal tract, which may be helpful for relieving indigestion, constipation, flatulence, and diarrhea. This could be especially helpful for those people with irritable bowel syndrome (IBS).
- **Parsley:** herb. Don't ignore this popular garnish; parsley is more than just a fancy plate decoration. It is good for healthy vision, the blood, and the heart because it contains high amounts of vitamins A, C, and K; folate; and iron. Research suggests parsley may act as a diuretic to decrease water retention and bloating.

Fact Stack

Shift your appetite clock. Eat less in the evening so you are hungrier in the morning. Research shows when we eat 70 percent of our calories in the early part of the day, we can lose 1.5 pounds more in six weeks than those who eat most of their calories in the evening.

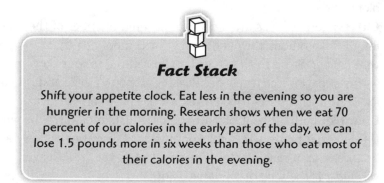

Fats, Oils, and Spreads

Fats undeniably add flavor and a rich texture to our food. Some fats are heart smart, while other fats cause ticker trouble. Here are my fat favorites.

Liquid Oils. If a fat is liquid at room temperature, it is a heart-healthy fat. Liquid oils include sesame, peanut, olive, flaxseed, sunflower, grape seed, almond, avocado, walnut, safflower, and others. On the other hand, fats that are solid at room temperature (butter, lard, stick margarine, partially hydrogenated shortening) have saturated or trans fats that are not good for healthy cholesterol levels. Among all your choices of healthy liquid oils, how do you decide which oils to use? Consider two things:

1. Smoke point—this is how much heat the oil can take before it starts smoking and tasting funky.
2. Oil flavor—do you want to impart a peanut, sesame, or olive flavor, or do you want something with less taste?

The smoke points vary depending on how the oil is processed, but in general:

- High-heat cooking (grilling, high-intensity stir-fry, and broiling): grape seed, peanut, safflower
- Medium-heat cooking (pan sauté and baking): canola, corn, olive, sesame, sunflower
- No direct heat (just to drizzle on cold or warm food): flaxseed oil

Olive oil has the reputation of being the healthy favorite, and although it has more heart-smart monounsaturated fat than almost all other oils, experiment with other liquid oils to add a variety of flavor to your food. As long as it is liquid at room temperature, an oil has healthy fats. I use all the oils but find I grab olive oil the most often. There are several types, such as extra virgin, virgin, and light (meaning less olive flavor, but not fewer calories!). But my favorite is cold-pressed *extra-virgin olive oil* since it is the least processed version, has the most olive flavor, and has the highest amount of healthy antioxidant compounds called polyphenols. No matter what type of fat you choose, healthy or unhealthy, use it sparingly because all fats have a waist-expanding 120 calories per tablespoon. For best taste quality, purchase oil in dark-tinted bottles, and store it out of direct light in a cool place.

Trans-Fat-Free Margarine. Butter has saturated fat, which raises bad LDL cholesterol, and stick margarine has trans fats, which also raise bad LDL cholesterol *and* decrease the good HDL cholesterol. What to spread? Use the healthy *trans-fat-free* margarines sold in tubs. They have about 45 to 80 calories per tablespoon, so still use them sparingly.

Sprays. Cans of cooking spray are just typical cooking oils that shoot out of the nozzle in a very fine mist with the help of compressed gas. There is nothing unhealthy about cooking spray; in fact, they are a great product for portioning out only a tiny amount of high-calorie oils. I like brands such as Spectrum because they use quality oils, organic grain alcohol from corn, and soy lecithin for a nice spraying consistency and ozone-friendly compressed gas. Use cooking spray when you want to prevent food from sticking on cookware or to keep spices from falling off foods you are going to cook. If you want a big flavor punch, put the spray can down and go to the regular oil in a bottle.

Olives. Olives contain a lot of fat, but about 75 percent of it is monounsaturated, or good, fat—a type that may reduce blood cholesterol levels and the risk of heart disease. In fact, researchers think that Mediterranean countries have lower rates of heart disease because olives and olive oil are key parts of the Mediterranean diet. Olives are also rich in vitamin E, iron, and fiber. They may even ease joint pain in people with arthritis because they contain polyphenols (a class of antioxidants) that decrease inflammation.

Avocados. Avocados are one fatty fruit—each 322-calorie avocado contains about 30 grams of fat, but 85 percent comes from the heart-healthy unsaturated types. Avocados contain more lutein (beneficial for eye health and vision) and the antioxidant vitamin E than almost

Craving Control

Enjoy social sweets only. Eating cakes, cookies, cupcakes, and pie always tastes better (and carries less guilt) when you are in a group rather than solo. Plus you're not likely to eat as much of that favorite sweet treat when you're in good company.

all other fruits. They also have a shockingly high amount of fiber—13.5 grams each (that's equivalent to the fiber in four to five bowls of oatmeal!). I put avocados in the condiment section (even though they technically are fruit) because they add a lot of flavor and creamy texture to many recipes.

Sweeteners

Humans are hardwired to like the sweet taste, so why fight our innate preference? We should include sweeteners in our diet—but in moderate amounts. As with all foods, I prefer to use sweeteners that have minimal processing to retain trace amounts of minerals and more healthy plant compounds. Your body probably doesn't notice much difference between processed sugar and more natural sugars, because they are all simple sugars without many measurable nutrients. Nonetheless, I still seek out the least processed of the lot.

Those little pink, blue, and yellow packets of artificial sweeteners are not dangerous, but here is my feeling: artificial sugar substitutes have an intense sweetness that can cause a "hyper sweet tooth." I have found that many people who overuse these fake sweeteners lose their ability to appreciate more subtle sweetness such as that in fresh fruit. I do not insist on taking them out of my clients' diets, but I think it is a good idea to use them only occasionally and to retrain the taste buds to find more joy in naturally sweet fruit and a drizzle of honey here and there.

The more natural types of sweeteners can be either dry and granular or syrupy like honey. Here are the ones I am sweet on.

Granulated Sugars. The regular white sugar you get in the store does start out as a natural plant product growing in fields as either sugarcane or sugar beets. Once the natural product gets through the processing and refining treatments, it does not resemble its original form in appearance or nutrition. All sugars are processed to some degree, but white and brown sugar are considered the most highly refined and processed (stripped of healthy minerals). The less processed, more natural sugars (which may have a trace amount of healthy plant minerals) include:

Demerara
Evaporated cane juice"
Muscovado (Barbados)
Rapadura
Sucanat ("sugarcane natural")
Turbinado

Syruplike Sweeteners. So sweet, just a dab will do ya. *Honey* might "bee" the newest health food on the block: research shows it contains antioxidants that may protect us against chronic diseases such as heart disease and cancer. Other health buzz about honey: it may boost our immune system by feeding good bacteria in the gut. Honey also has antibacterial properties and can be applied topically to heal skin wounds. Seriously, how amazing is that?

I don't think I had a drop of *real maple syrup* in my life until I recently went to a nutrition conference in Quebec, Canada, the maple syrup capital of the world. I now use maple syrup as my primary sweetener on things like sweet potatoes, pancakes, and yogurt. Grade A syrup is lighter in flavor (in light, medium, and dark versions), and Grade B has a very dark, robust flavor.

Agave (uh-GAH-vee) *nectar* is a sweet syrup that comes from the agave plant (which is not a cactus but rather a succulent similar to the aloe vera). Agave has what I call a "health halo," meaning it is considered so healthy that many overportion it. This sweet nectar is a natural product, but it still has 60 calories per tablespoon (20 calories per teaspoon), so use it sparingly. It is sweeter and thinner than honey and has a delicate flavor. It goes well in any recipe you want to taste sweet without the stronger flavors of honey or maple syrup. It also blends well in hot and cold beverages such as iced tea and coffee.

Two other sticky sweet and satisfying choices include *brown rice syrup* and *barley malt syrup*. I have at least one of those in my fridge for a little sweet variety. The brown rice syrup is very mild, and the barley malt syrup tastes hearty, almost like deep, nutty molasses.

Chocolate. Dark chocolate, also known as semisweet or bitter-sweet, is considered healthier than milk chocolate because it's made with more cocoa beans and less sugar. Cocoa beans contain plant compounds called flavonoids, which may lower cholesterol and blood pressure and increase blood flow to the brain to keep our memory sharp. Look for chocolate that is made without added milk fat (check the ingredient list to make sure milk fat is not listed). Choose chocolate that has at least 35 percent cocoa, but higher percentages such as 60 or 70 percent are even better because they have more healthy cocoa beans, less sugar, and a stronger chocolate taste. Purchase natural cocoa powder rather than Dutch-processed, as the processing decreases the healthy antioxidant properties of cocoa.

Ready-to-Eat Condiments

Classic and quick condiments definitely have a place in your cooking. Just choose them carefully by looking at the labels and investigating ingredients. The following are my favorites along with guidelines on how to find some of your own.

Craving Control

Adopt the no-free-sweets rule. If cookies are just sitting out in your office free for the taking, tell yourself that if you really want a cookie you can go to a coffee shop and *buy* yourself one. Buying a goodie is extra effort and will reduce the number of sweets you eat.

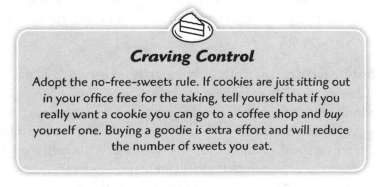

Ketchup and Mustard. This is the all-American condiment duo. A tablespoon of ketchup is about 15 to 20 calories, and I like brands such as Heinz organic or Annie's Naturals, which are sweetened with sugar instead of high-fructose corn syrup (HFCS). Our bodies probably don't know the difference between HFCS and sugar, because they are processed in similar ways, but I still seek out products without HFCS. A tablespoon of mustard, about 5 calories or less, adds a nice zip to sandwiches, and I use it in all of my homemade salad-dressing recipes as a tangy thickener.

Barbecue Sauce. This sweet and tangy condiment is my favorite. Choose a brand that has less than 50 calories and fewer than 250 milligrams sodium per 2 tablespoons, such as Annie's Naturals (I also like this brand because it is sweetened with natural brown rice syrup instead of HFCS).

Eggless Mayonnaise. I like the taste of eggless mayo from companies such as Spectrum and Nasoya. If you don't choose the vegetarian eggless version, choose light mayo or light sandwich spread (e.g., Miracle Whip). *Aioli*, a fancy term for flavored mayonnaise, is a fun condiment you can make yourself with any type of herbs and seasonings. Horseradish and lemon stirred into mayo is one of my favorite aioli formulas!

Low-Fat Sour Cream. As with most dairy products, you can get this made from cow's milk or soy milk. Choose low-fat versions to save about 10 calories and 1 gram of saturated fat for every tablespoon. If you do choose a soy version, check the label to see that it has no hydrogenated oil.

Salad Dressing. I never thought I would be a person to go through the time and trouble of making my own salad dressing. Stores have hundreds of premade options, and many of them are healthy choices. However, I wanted to make a flaxseed oil dressing to get omega-3 fatty acids for heart health and skin moisture. (Omega-3 fats help keep skin moist from the inside, which is a great antiaging beauty trick.) My husband and I both think the taste of my Universal Lemon-Flax Vinaigrette (see Index) is worth the effort of making it ourselves. Just as a reminder, you shouldn't cook with flaxseed oil, but you can put it on warm foods. So in addition to using it on cold salads, you can try this dressing on cooked vegetables, fish, and chicken.

When you do buy premade salad dressing (which I still do on occasion), check for labels where 2 tablespoons have less than 90 calories, 1 gram or less saturated fat, and less than 240 milligrams of sodium.

Vinegars. Vinegar's tart and tangy flavor makes a great salad or fruit topping with 0 to 15 calories per tablespoon. My favorites are red wine, rice, balsamic, and white balsamic vinegar. I use white balsamic when I want the sweet flavor of balsamic vinegar without the dark brown color. In most salad dressing recipes, you will typically see a ratio of about two or three parts oil to one part vinegar, but I make salad dressings with more vinegar (two parts vinegar to only one part oil) to keep the calories down. For variety, try flavored vinegars such as fig, raspberry, or pear.

Canned Tomatoes and Salsa. Canned tomato products contain a compound called lycopene (LY-ko-peen), an antioxidant that may protect us against heart disease and some types of cancer such as prostate, ovarian, and lung. The healthy lycopene content of a fresh tomato increases when it is cooked or canned. To best absorb lycopene, eat it with food that contains a little fat, such as cheese or olive oil.

You can quickly make your own pasta sauce, to save calories, sodium, and money—just sauté your favorite no-salt-added canned tomatoes with a little garlic, Italian seasoning, and a splash of balsamic vinegar (my secret ingredient). Wow, is that a good pasta sauce! When you buy canned tomato products, look for no-salt-added versions.

I also buy jars of prepared pasta sauce and read the product labels to find those with less than 80 calories and less than 500 milligrams sodium per ½ cup serving. My favorites have around 350 milligrams of sodium per ½ cup serving.

Salsa fits into all of this tomato talk. It is a healthy, high-flavor condiment with a low calorie count—only 10 calories for 2 tablespoons. Find brands that have less than 150 milligrams of sodium per serving,

Time Crunch

Read labels fast, using the 5 and 20 rule. When you see a *5 percent* in the right-hand column labeled "percent DV," the food is *low* in that nutrient. When you see *20 percent,* it is *high* in that nutrient.

which is the sodium equivalent of just one pinch of salt. Here's my salsa suggestion: Buy it. Use it. Period.

Sprinkle Me Healthy

There are three things that you can shake on your food for flavor and nutrition: flaxseeds, nutritional yeast, and seaweed.

Flax Sprinkle. Flaxseeds have earned superstardom status in the Flex world because of their high alpha-linolenic-acid content, an omega-3 fatty acid that may help with arthritis and the prevention of heart disease, high blood pressure, high cholesterol, and some types of cancer. Fish is very high in omega-3 fatty acids, but for those who don't eat their 12 ounces of fish (two fish meals) per week, flaxseeds are a way to get similar health benefits. Flaxseeds must be *ground* to grant the most health benefits, so you can buy the whole seeds and grind your own (in a coffee grinder) or purchase already ground flaxseeds, also called flax meal.

The easiest way to eat ground flaxseeds is to keep them in a clean, Parmesan cheese shaker that you can buy at a container store. Having them ready-to-shake, straight from the fridge makes it so easy to sprinkle on cereal, yogurt, oatmeal, salads, and stir-fries. Aim for about 1 to 2 tablespoons of the *ground flaxseeds* per day (37 calories and 2 grams of fiber per tablespoon) or about one tablespoon of flaxseed *oil* per day (120 calories per tablespoon.) My Universal Lemon-Flax Vinaigrette recipe (see Index) has flaxseed oil as the base. You can get flaxseeds and flax oil in many grocery stores and in health food stores, usually in or near the supplement department.

Nutritional Yeast Sprinkle. You can find nutritional yeast (not brewer's yeast) in health food stores, usually in the supplement section. It is a great source of vegetarian protein and vitamin B_{12}. It usually comes in big containers, so keep some in a clean Parmesan cheese shaker, which makes it is easier to use. It tastes very similar to Parmesan, but every 2 tablespoons of nutritional yeast has 2 grams less fat, 4 times more fiber, double the protein of the cheese, and 133 percent of your daily B_{12}. Here are the nutrition stats for 2 tablespoons of nutritional yeast: 60 calories, 1 gram fat, 4 grams fiber, 8 grams protein, 8 micrograms B_{12} (133 percent daily needs), and 9.6 milligrams riboflavin (565 percent daily needs).

Seaweed Sprinkle. Sea vegetables are a world of wonder, excitement, and good nutrition. Sea vegetables (or seaweed) are plants that grow underwater. They contain healthy minerals such as iodine, iron, magnesium, calcium, and phosphorus. My preferred seaweed sprinkle, made of sesame seeds, seaweed, and sea salt, is Seaweed Gomasio by Eden foods (edenfoods.com). Each teaspoon has three types of sea vegetables (dulse, nori, and kombu), only 15 calories, and thirty times less sodium than salt, so it is a great low-sodium salt replacement. This has lots of umami—savory meatlike flavor—perfect for elevating vegetarian dishes a few culinary octaves.

Craving Control

Determine your hunger location. Eat when your stomach is hungry, not according to your mind or mouth. If you feel a craving for something, this is located in your *mind*. If you have a taste for something, this is located in your *mouth*. If you have a light, empty feeling in your *stomach*, that is true physical hunger and indicates the right time to eat.

Beverages

As my husband says, "Water is the giver of life." I couldn't agree more. Every life-sustaining body process needs water to function. It helps transport oxygen and nutrients throughout your body, maintain a proper body temperature, keep your mental focus, lubricate joints, and remove waste. The Institute of Medicine of the National Academies recommends that women should drink about 9 glasses (72 ounces) and men about 12 glasses (96 ounces) of fluids each day.

You don't have to drink just plain water, but beware of extra calories that can sneak into your cup. Gourmet coffee drinks, juices, smoothies, and soda can add up to hundreds of excess, gut-busting calories each day. Don't buy soda frequently; just have it as a very occasional treat. A study in the July 2007 issue of *Circulation* (journal from the American Heart Association) found people who drink one or more sodas per day (regular *or diet*) have a 31 percent increased risk of becoming obese compared to people who drank little to no soda.

My favorite drinks are calorie free but still have some flavor, as flavored fluids encourage us to drink more:

- **Water:** flat or sparkling with my own natural flavor enhancements such as lemon, lime, orange, cucumber, or mint.
- **Coffee:** may decrease risk of diabetes by 30 percent and enhance memory and performance. Only about two to three cups a day (8 ounces each) is recommended to keep caffeine in check—too much caffeine can lead to anxiety, sleep issues, irritability, irregular heartbeat, and jitters. Caffeine's half-life (or amount of time it takes for half of the chemical to leave your body) is six hours, so if you drink it late in the afternoon it *will* affect your sleep (even if you think it doesn't). Keep coffee to a morning perk-me-up, and go decaf in the later parts of the day.
- **Tea:** green, black, and white tea all come from the same plant and just differ on how they are processed. They all contain powerful compounds such as catechins (KA-teh-kins), which may help us burn up to 67 extra calories each day, prevent cavities, and prevent some cancers such as skin, esophagus, and stomach. Since tea has about three times less caffeine than coffee (30 mg per cup of tea

Craving Control

Start a tea tradition. Drink a cup of dessert-flavored tea such as English toffee or white chocolate macadamia nut after meals. Tea has zero calories and promotes a healthy heart.

versus 100 mg per cup of coffee), it is a more responsible way to caffeinate throughout the entire day. Types of decaf tea include red tea, called *rooibos* (pronounced ROY-bus); *herbal* teas, such as mint, apple cinnamon, and chamomile; and *roasted barley* tea, which has a deep nutty, almost coffeelike flavor. Fruit-flavored teas can be herbal (decaf), or fruit flavor can be added to caffeinated tea. Just read the label to see which contain caffeine. Steep your tea for four minutes to release the most health benefits, and aim to drink about three cups (24 ounces) per day, which is the typical amount consumed in Asian countries.

If you choose to drink alcoholic beverages, moderation is key. Moderate amounts of wine, beer, and hard alcohol may *all* have health benefits such as decreased risk of heart disease, but there are still some people who should not drink, such as pregnant women, those with a history of breast cancer, and people taking medications that react negatively with alcohol. Moderation by definition is one drink per day for a woman and two per day for a man. (And no, you can't save up your daily quota for a one-night drinking binge!) One drink is 12 ounces of regular or light beer, 5 ounces of wine, or a 1.5-ounce shot (jigger) of hard alcohol.

Choose drinks in the 100-calorie or less range, such as a 12-ounce light beer, a 5-ounce glass of wine, or a shot of the hard stuff in club soda (not tonic water, because it has calories); other mixers, froufrou drinks, and blended concoctions can have more than 500 calories each. Here's an example: if you are at a Mexican fiesta, say no thank you (manners, manners) to the 500-calorie margarita and opt for a

Fact Stack

Downsize your dinnerware. We rely on visual cues such as bowl, plate, and utensil size to help gauge portions. We eat 31 percent more food when using a large bowl instead of a smaller one and 14.5 percent more when using a large spoon rather than a smaller one.

100-calorie Corona light with a lime. Even though your drink has only 100 calories, you have to beware the *alcohol munchies.* Just a few sips of alcohol can increase your appetite and cause you to make unhealthy food choices and take overzealous portions! A great tip is to delay your drinking until the middle or end of a meal. Then many of your food decisions have already been made, plus the longer you delay, the less time you have to accidentally overindulge. My favorite drink is a wine spritzer of 2.5 ounces of wine with 5 ounces of club soda for a grand total of just 50 calories.

Flex Fundamentals Group 5: Sugar and Spice (and Everything in Between) Summary

- Condiments can make or break your healthy eating plan. Stock up on and prepare healthy, flavorful condiments to make your foods go from blah to ta-dah!
- Keep your rack filled with the baker's dozen (thirteen) best herbs and spices.
- Each week, have two to three fresh herbs wrapped in a towel burrito in your fridge.
- Healthy fats and sweeteners are delicious diet additions and can be healthy if chosen wisely.
- Carefully chosen, ready-to-eat condiments such as ketchup, mustard, barbecue sauce, mayo, sour cream, canned tomatoes, and salsa are convenient to have on hand.

- You can shake and sprinkle your way to health with flaxseeds, nutritional yeast, and sea vegetables (the upscale way to say *seaweed*).
- Drink to your newfound healthier flexitarian lifestyle by choosing beverages that are lightly flavored but don't weigh you down with excess calories.

Fact Stack

Food is the best source of vitamins and minerals; however, adults who are trying to lose weight should take a basic daily multiple vitamin and mineral supplement to ensure they get all of their nutrients while decreasing calories. Women should choose a multivitamin for women, because they are tailored to meet women's higher iron needs. Men should choose a multivitamin for men, which will have little to no iron.

Fill in the Nutrient Gaps from A to Z (Vitamin A to Zinc)

Meat is an optional rather than a mandatory part of the human diet. Many vegetarians feel like they have to eat meat every now and again just to get "the nutrition from meat." It is possible to get 100 percent balanced and adequate nutrition from plant foods (although vegans who eat absolutely no animal products may need a B_{12} supplement). This is a flexitarian book, so I am not suggesting you shouldn't eat meat. Rather, I am suggesting you should enjoy meat as part of a meaningful meat event, in fun social situations, as a culinary experience, or for reasons other than thinking you *have* to eat it for nutrition—because you don't.

Although it is possible to get all of your nutrition from plants, there are 10 nutrients vegetarians should pay attention to including vitamin A, calcium, vitamin D, B_{12}, riboflavin, omega-3 fatty acid, iodine, protein, iron, and zinc. Here is a basic four-point checklist to ensure that you are meeting those ten specific nutrient needs:

- ☐ Eat *orange and green produce* regularly for vitamin A.
- ☐ Drink *milk or fortified soy milk* regularly for quick calcium, vitamin D, B_{12}, and riboflavin.
- ☐ Shake *ground flaxseeds* on your cereal, yogurt, and salads, or use *flaxseed oil* (such as my Universal Lemon-Flax Vinaigrette [see Index]) on raw or cooked foods for omega-3 fatty acids.
- ☐ Include *plant proteins* such beans and lentils to meet your protein, iron, and zinc needs.

Note: Vegans may want to consider taking a B_{12} supplement or regularly sprinkling a vegetarian formula of nutritional yeast on food (tastes like Parmesan cheese).

Part Three

Five-Week Flex Meal Plan and Five-Main-Ingredient Flex Recipes

If you are ready to embrace Flex recipes, you are in the right part of the book. This part contains the five-main-ingredient recipes organized into five weeks of meal plans with corresponding weekly *shopping lists*. Each recipe makes *one serving*, but each also can easily be multiplied to feed as many people as necessary.

These recipes have been tested and approved by my family, friends, clients, and cooking-class participants. I make these recipes because they are quick, nutritious, and great tasting. In total, there are thirty-five breakfast recipes, thirty-five lunches, thirty-five dinners, and thirty-five different snacks. You can follow the plan week by week as outlined, or in the flexitarian spirit you can switch and swap recipes and make a plan that is more personalized to your tastes and preferences.

Here are some fun features of my Flex meals and recipes:

- **Mix and match:** The meals and snacks can be mixed and matched because this plan is based on my *3-4-5* meal plan system: each of the thirty-five breakfast choices are around *300* calories, each of the lunches are *400* calories, and every dinner is *500* calories (instead of being as easy as 1, 2, 3 . . . this meal plan is as easy as 3, 4, 5!). Each of the thirty-five different snacks are about 150 calories, and if you choose two, a day's calories add up to about 1,500—the perfect amount for losing weight without sacrificing satisfaction. Depending on your activity level, gender, height, and weight, you may need slightly more calories or less. If you are losing too slowly, pay more attention to portions, and if you are losing too fast or feel too hungry, add a snack or an extra portion at the meal when you are the hungriest.

  If you love variety, each week's Flex meal plan offers enough recipes to eat something different every day. If you prefer more of a routine, just pick a few favorite meals and snacks and repeat them. Look over a specific week's meal plan and pick one or two of your favorite breakfasts, two to three lunches, two to three dinners, and two different snacks. You should be trying plenty of new things, although experimenting with too many new recipes can

Fact Stack

The Centers for Disease Control and Prevention (CDC) estimates that the average woman eats 1,877 calories per day and the average man eats 2,618 calories per day. Based on those averages, women need 1,200 to 1,500 calories per day for weight loss, and men need closer to 1,800 to 2,000. This Flex eating plan is 1,500 calories per day, which is a good place for most people to start. If you would prefer a 1,200-calorie plan, omit the snacks. For an 1,800-calorie plan, double the portion at breakfast (600 calories instead of 300 calories).

be energy and time-consuming. This is a life plan, so you have a lifetime to try the 140 recipes. Have fun, and enjoy all of your tasty explorations.

- **Flex Swap:** I have added the Flex Swap feature to many recipes. Flex Swaps are suggestions for recipe alterations and ingredient exchanges, such as how to add chicken, turkey, fish, or red meat to a vegetarian recipe. Look for the Flex Swap icon for ingredient substitutions throughout the recipes and meal plans. The swaps will only slightly change the nutrition information. You can use the given original recipe nutrition facts as an estimate when using a Flex Swap.
- **Nutrition information:** I have included the nutrition information for all of these disease-fighting, plant-based recipes. In addition to being calorie controlled, each main dish or meal meets the American Heart Association's heart-check-mark certification for sodium (less than 720–960 mg) and saturated fat (less than 6–8 g). Plus, the recipes contain no artificial ingredients such as trans fat, high-fructose corn syrup, or sugar substitutes. Mmmm—naturally wholesome, filling, and delicious!
- **Shopping lists:** The weekly shopping lists will save you time in the grocery store. They are set up for one person, but you can easily multiply the ingredients if you are cooking for more than one. You can buy everything on the list to make all the meals and snacks, or just check off the items you need to make the recipes that interest you. You can photocopy the page and bring it to the store with you, or you can go to my website, dawnjacksonblatner.com, and download copies of the shopping lists. If you come across an ingredient on the list or in a recipe that you don't recognize or want to learn more about, refer to Part Two, Five Flex Food Groups.

These flexitarian meals are not "diet" food. There are plenty of über-low-calorie, fake food recipes out there that have zero taste and will leave you scavenging through the cabinets for snacks all night. If you are looking for that, you will not find it here. Flex recipes are brimming with fat (the healthy kind), carbs (the right kind), protein, and enough salt to bring out the flavor in your food. They are *real* food and are not

Fact Stack

Follow the Flex meal plan. Research shows that people who follow a structured eating plan for six months lose about 26.5 pounds, whereas people who try to lose weight not following a meal plan lose less.

made with artificial chemicals and ingredients. The easy-to-prepare (fast and simple) recipes are filling and satisfying. As you become more comfortable with the recipes, experiment by changing and tweaking them: add a different herb or spice, try an alternative type of bean, or exchange a vegetable or fruit with something else you have on hand.

Flex Fridge, Pantry, and Spice Rack Staples

These are the must-have ingredients for your fridge, pantry, and spice rack that are used consistently in many of the Flex recipes and weekly Flex meal plans. Before you begin trying all of the delicious Flex recipes, make sure you have these basic *fridge*, *pantry*, and *spice rack* staples on hand. There is also a checklist of essential Flex kitchen tools that make preparing meals more efficient.

Fridge

1. Barbecue sauce
2. Ketchup and mustard
3. Lemons and limes
4. Milk: skim or soy milk
5. Salsa: red, green, or both
6. Universal Lemon-Flax Vinaigrette. Make this each week, and keep it on hand because it is used in many of the recipes and is a great way to get your heart-healthy omega-3 fatty acids. Buy an empty squeeze ketchup bottle from a container store, and keep the dressing in your fridge to use over the course of a week (it lasts about seven days or so in the fridge).

Pantry

1. Canned tomatoes (no salt added): diced, crushed, and sauce
2. Cooking spray
3. Garlic
4. Honey
5. Maple syrup
6. Oils: olive, sesame, and peanut
7. Onions
8. Vanilla extract
9. Vinegar: rice, balsamic, and white balsamic
10. Nut butters: peanut butter, almond butter, and sunflower seed butter

Universal Lemon-Flax Vinaigrette

Makes 6 servings (2 tablespoons each)

¼ cup lemon juice (juice from 1 to 2 lemons)
¼ cup flaxseed oil
¼ cup white balsamic vinegar
1 tablespoon Dijon mustard
1 clove garlic, minced
Salt and black pepper to taste

Whisk all ingredients together. Keep in fridge about seven days.

Nutrition Info (2 tablespoons): 88 calories, 9 g total fat, 1 g saturated fat, 0 mg cholesterol, 59 mg sodium, 2 g carbohydrates, 0 g fiber, 0 g protein

Your Baker's Dozen Spice Rack

1. Buttermilk ranch seasoning
2. Chili powder
3. Cinnamon
4. Crushed, red chili-pepper flakes
5. Cumin (ground)
6. Curry powder
7. Italian seasoning
8. Old Bay
9. Smoky paprika
10. Pie spice: apple or pumpkin
11. Salt and black pepper
12. Rosemary
13. Sage

Essential Flex Kitchen Tools Checklist

Having the right kitchen tools is essential for easy preparation of healthy flexitarian meals. You don't have to break the bank buying gadgets or clutter your counters with fancy food equipment that you don't know how to use and don't want to clean. Here is the basic must-have Flex kitchen tools checklist:

- ☐ **10- to 12-inch nonstick sauté pan.** I use this every day. Make sure it is oven safe in case you want to pop it under the broiler.
- ☐ **2-quart saucepan.** You will use this to cook all of your whole grains, such as brown rice, quinoa, and whole-grain pasta.
- ☐ **2-quart glass or ceramic oven-safe casserole dish.**
- ☐ **8-quart stockpot or soup pot.** This is for larger batches of soups and whole grains.
- ☐ **Can opener.** Nothing fancy, just something to open the countless cans of beans that flexitarians eat!
- ☐ **Cheese grater.** This is also useful for grating veggies such as zucchini, eggplant, and onions to toss into frittatas, enchiladas, or potato hash.
- ☐ **Citrus press.** Fresh-squeezed lemon, lime, and orange juice add bright, fresh flavor to food.
- ☐ **Colander.** This is for rinsing canned beans and draining whole-wheat pasta.

Out and About

Decrease your dining-out frequency. People who lose weight and keep it off successfully dine out no more than two to three times per week in restaurants and less than once per week at fast-food joints.

Craving Control

Three magic words: ask yourself, *"Am I hungry?"* before eating anything. It is a quick way to be more connected to what is causing you to reach mindlessly for food.

- ☐ **Cookie sheet with sides (jelly-roll pan).** I would get two. I don't make cookies on these, but I use them to roast large batches of veggies such as onions, potatoes, parsnips, cauliflower, carrots, fennel bulb, butternut squash fries, brussels sprouts, and so on.
- ☐ **Cutting board.** I like my Epicurean brand cutting board (visit epicurious.com), which is made of eco-friendly wood fibers and is dishwasher safe.
- ☐ **Garlic press.** Garlic has more health benefits when it is crushed or minced well—a press can do this better than hand chopping.
- ☐ **Grill pan.** If you don't have a grill or it is too cold, rainy, or snowy to go outside, an indoor grill pan is next best. I prefer rectangular ones without handles, with grill grooves on one side and a smooth, griddle for pancakes on the other.
- ☐ **Hand blender with attachments.** This is also called an immersion blender and is my absolute favorite kitchen tool. Get the one with the *chopper* attachment, which turns it into a mini food processor. It is a great kitchen gadget to make the best flexitarian dips, sauces, spreads, creamy soups, and desserts with very little cleanup. You could also use a regular blender or food processor if you are cooking for a larger crowd. I use Braun, but many brands are available.
- ☐ **High-heat rubber spatula.** Get two of these. I use them to stir and sauté everything.
- ☐ **Measuring cups.** You will need these for both wet and dry ingredients. Wet measuring cups usually have a spout, and dry cups are usually sold in packs of six ranging from ¼ to 1 cup.

- ☐ **Measuring spoons.** These are especially important for measuring oil. At 120 calories per tablespoon, oil is one of the most important things to measure when cooking.
- ☐ **Mixing bowls.** I like glass ones with lids; you can use these for mixing and tossing and storing foods like salads.
- ☐ **Paring knife.** This is a good knife for small work, such as avocados or apples.
- ☐ **Santoku 5- to 7-inch knife.** Chop, slice, mince, dice—this knife style provides comfortable control and excellent cutting performance. I use this knife every day.
- ☐ **Storage bags and containers.** Plastic sandwich bags and all sizes of resealable containers are Flex kitchen must-haves for storing extras and transporting healthy snacks and lunches.
- ☐ **Tongs with high-heat plastic edges.** These are good for grilling, tossing salads, and sautéing.

Time Crunch

Design a dinner deck of cards. Write down five to seven family-favorite dinners on index cards—the front has the recipe name and the back has the ingredients. Keep this deck of dinner ideas in your purse or car, and refer to it when grocery shopping so you don't forget key ingredients.

Week One Recipes, Meal Plan, Shopping List

Week One Flex Breakfasts

Fig and Flax Oatmeal

I love figs so much that a friend bought me dried figs shaped into a huge salami log for Christmas one year! Anything with dried figs reminds me of Fig Newton cookies—yum.

- ½ cup skim milk or soy milk
- ½ cup water
- ½ cup rolled oats
- 2 dried figs, chopped
- 1 tablespoon ground flaxseeds
- 1 teaspoon honey

Bring milk, water, and oats to a boil. Simmer and stir for 5 minutes. Add figs, flaxseeds, and honey.

297 calories, 6 g total fat, 1 g saturated fat, 2 mg cholesterol, 61 mg sodium, 52 g carbohydrates, 8 g fiber, 12 g protein

Craving Control

Indulge in a supersized, adult raisinette. Dip a dried fig into melted dark chocolate.

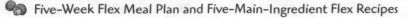

Swiss Apple Muesli

Muesli was introduced around 1900 by a Swiss doctor named Maximilian Bircher-Benner who treated his patients primarily with a diet rich in fresh fruit and vegetables. This breakfast is close to the doctor's original: rolled oats, a grated apple, and nuts.

½ cup rolled oats
½ cup skim milk or soy milk
½ small apple, finely chopped
1 tablespoon sliced almonds
1 teaspoon honey

Mix *raw* oats with milk. Stir in apple, almonds, and honey. Let sit 10 minutes or overnight in the fridge.

291 calories, 7 g total fat, 1 g saturated fat, 2 mg cholesterol, 54 mg sodium, 47 g carbohydrates, 6 g fiber, 12 g protein

Fact Stack

Eat an apple a day to keep hunger at bay. Eating an apple about 15 minutes before a meal can help you eat about 190 calories less at the meal.

Apricot-Almond Brown Rice Breakfast

Rise and shine with brown rice instead of just thinking about it for dinner. Chopped apricots and almonds give it a delicately sweet morning attitude.

¾ cup cooked brown rice (precooked microwavable or leftover)
3 dried apricots, chopped
2 tablespoons sliced almonds
1 teaspoon maple syrup

Top warm brown rice with apricots, almonds, and maple syrup.

300 calories, 7 g total fat, 1 g saturated fat, 0 mg cholesterol, 4 mg sodium, 54 g carbohydrates, 6 g fiber, 7 g protein

Italian Onion and Potato Omelet

The ingredients are perfect for meat-eaters or vegetarians craving a hearty, hot, and savory way to start the day. This also makes a great dinner or brunch dish.

- ¼ small onion, diced
- ½ small potato (with skin), grated
- ¼ cup vegetarian crumbles (sausage style)
- 1 tablespoon Italian seasoning
- Cooking spray
- 1 whole egg + 2 egg whites, beaten
- 1 small orange

In a pan sprayed with cooking spray, sauté onion, potato, crumbles, and Italian seasoning over medium-high heat for 5 minutes. Add eggs and cook for 3 to 4 minutes; flip and cook an additional 2 minutes. Serve with orange on the side.

286 calories, 7 g total fat, 2 g saturated fat, 212 mg cholesterol, 310 mg sodium, 36 g carbohydrates, 8 g fiber, 22 g protein

Flex Swap ¼ cup vegetarian sausage-style crumbles for 1 ounce cooked, diced low-fat chicken sausage.

Banana-Pecan Waffles

I create diets for national magazines, and waffles are always among the readers' favorite meals. I included several waffle breakfasts in this book to please all of the waffle lovers—not to mention that whole-grain frozen waffles are a superfast breakfast.

2 frozen whole-grain waffles
½ small banana, sliced
1 tablespoon chopped pecans
1 teaspoon maple syrup

Toast waffles. Top with banana, pecans, and a drizzle of syrup.

311 calories, 14 g total fat, 2 g saturated fat, 0 mg cholesterol, 330 mg sodium, 42 g carbohydrates, 4 g fiber, 7 g protein

Granola-Berry Parfait

Basic parfait with a portioning trick of mine: use a crushed granola bar instead of portioning your own granola from a whole box—granola genius!

1 cup unsweetened mixed frozen berries, thawed
1 container (6 ounces) low-fat plain yogurt
1 whole-grain crunchy granola bar, crumbled

Layer berries, yogurt, and crumbled granola bar.

299 calories, 3 g total fat, 0 g saturated fat, 3 mg cholesterol, 203 mg sodium, 57 g carbohydrates, 8 g fiber, 13 g protein

Herbed Cheese and Tomato Bagel

This herbed cheese is made from whipped low-fat cottage cheese, which makes this a low-fat, high-protein spread or vegetable dip. The herbed cheese also can be stirred into cooked whole-wheat pasta as a fresh and creamy sauce. Drain the cottage cheese for a thicker spread.

½ cup low-fat cottage cheese
2 teaspoons chopped fresh chives
2 teaspoons chopped fresh parsley
2 teaspoons chopped fresh basil
Dash of black pepper
1 small whole-grain bagel, toasted
2 thick tomato slices

Blend cottage cheese with hand blender. Stir in fresh herbs and black pepper. Spread on toasted bagel, and top with tomato.

291 calories, 2 g total fat, 1 g saturated fat, 5 mg cholesterol, 370 mg sodium, 46 g carbohydrates, 4 g fiber, 22 g protein

Note: Whipped low-fat cottage cheese is a good substitute for cream cheese. Fat-free cream cheese has artificial colors, flavors, and preservatives and doesn't have much taste. The original, reduced-fat, and even light cream cheeses all have a hefty dose of unhealthy saturated fat.

Week One Flex Lunches

Caprese Pita

Tomatoes, basil, and fresh mozzarella taste great stuffed into a whole-grain pita. I prefer a pita to bread at lunchtime, because its pockets can hold lots of veggies.

- 1 ounce fresh mozzarella, chopped
- 1 cup halved cherry tomatoes
- ¼ cup chopped fresh basil
- 1 tablespoon pine nuts
- 2 tablespoons Universal Lemon-Flax Vinaigrette (see Index) or low-fat Italian dressing
- 1 whole-grain pita pocket, cut in half

Mix mozzarella, tomatoes, basil, pine nuts, and dressing together. Stuff mixture into pita halves.

406 calories, 21 g total fat, 5 g saturated fat, 15 mg cholesterol, 434 mg sodium, 43 g carbohydrates, 9 g fiber, 17 g protein

Note: Fresh mozzarella is usually packed in water and is softer than typical mozzarella with a delicate flavor.

Flex Swap 1 ounce mozzarella for ¼ cup white beans, rinsed and drained.

Fact Stack

Eat four to five times per day. People who are most successful at losing weight and keeping it off eat an average of four to five times per day, which translates into three meals and one snack, or three meals and two snacks.

Avocado and Black Bean Wraps

I eat this for lunch at least once a week because it is fast and flavorful.

- ¾ cup canned black beans, rinsed, drained, and smashed with fork
- ¼ avocado, chopped
- ¼ cup salsa
- ½ teaspoon cumin
- 1 lime, juiced
- 2 small (6-inch) whole-grain tortillas

Mix smashed beans, avocado, salsa, cumin, and lime juice. Wrap mixture in tortillas.

409 calories, 9 g total fat, 1 g saturated fat, 0 mg cholesterol, 437 mg sodium, 70 g carbohydrates, 19 g fiber, 18 g protein

Flex Swap ½ cup of black beans for 2 ounces cooked, diced chicken breast.

Artichoke and Tomato Panzella Salad

This hearty Italian salad made with bread is easy enough for lunch and delicious enough to bring to a party.

3 canned (in water) artichoke hearts, drained and chopped
½ cup halved cherry tomatoes
¾ cup canned cannellini beans, rinsed and drained
1 slice whole-grain bread, toasted and cut into bite-sized pieces
2 tablespoons Universal Lemon-Flax Vinaigrette (see Index) or low-fat Italian dressing
3 cups green spring salad mix

Mix artichokes, tomatoes, beans, toast pieces, and vinaigrette together. Put on top of salad greens.

404 calories, 11 g total fat, 1 g saturated fat, 0 mg cholesterol, 423 mg sodium, 61 g carbohydrates, 17 g fiber, 20 g protein

Flex Swap ½ cup of cannellini beans for 2 ounces (about 9 medium) frozen cooked shrimp, thawed.

All-American Burger

Classic ketchup, mustard, tomato, lettuce, and pickle make you want to burst into a few verses of "God Bless America."

1 frozen vegetarian burger, heated
1 whole-grain hamburger bun
1 slice cheddar cheese
1 tablespoon ketchup
1 teaspoon mustard
Lettuce and tomato slices
1 small apple

Put hot burger on bun and top with cheese, ketchup, mustard, lettuce, and tomato. Serve with apple.

404 calories, 14 g total fat, 7 g saturated fat, 28 mg cholesterol, 722 mg sodium, 49 g carbohydrates, 10 g fiber, 23 g protein

Flex Swap 1 slice cheddar cheese for ¼ avocado or 1 slice of vegetarian cheese.

Micro-Bean Burrito

Micro is short for *microwave*. Microwaving is one of my favorite ways to cook because it is so convenient.

¾ cup canned low-fat or vegetarian refried beans
2 small (6-inch) whole-grain tortillas
1 slice cheddar cheese, cut in half
¼ cup salsa
¾ cup romaine lettuce

Place beans in microwave-safe bowl and heat in microwave. Spread beans on tortillas, and top with cheese, salsa, and lettuce.

419 calories, 11 g total fat, 6 g saturated fat, 28 mg cholesterol, 699 mg sodium, 70 g carbohydrates, 12 g fiber, 23 g protein

Flex Swap 1 slice cheddar cheese for ¼ avocado or 1 slice of vegetarian cheese.

Fact Stack

In general, the longer vegetables are cooked, the more nutrients are lost. Microwaving is a quick-cooking method, so it keeps vegetables from losing valuable vitamins.

Red Grape and Walnut Salad

The dynamic duo of grapes and walnuts is popular at many restaurants. The special thing here is the addition of edamame.

- ½ cup red grapes, halved
- ¼ cup chopped walnuts
- ⅓ cup frozen edamame (shelled green soybeans), thawed
- 2 tablespoons Universal Lemon-Flax Vinaigrette (see Index) or low-fat Italian dressing
- 3 cups green spring salad mix

Toss all ingredients together.

410 calories, 31 g total fat, 3 g saturated fat, 0 mg cholesterol, 105 mg sodium, 29 g carbohydrates, 8 g fiber, 12 g protein

Flex Swap ⅓ cup edamame for 1½ ounces cooked, diced chicken breast.

Indian Lentil Wraps

Curry powder contains potent disease-fighting compounds such as curcumin, which may help heart health and cancer prevention and fight arthritis and Alzheimer's disease. This is a delicious way to prevent disease.

- ¾ cup canned lentils, rinsed and drained
- ½ teaspoon curry powder
- 2 tablespoons raisins
- ¾ cup shredded carrots
- 2 small (6-inch) whole-grain tortillas

Mix lentils, curry powder, raisins, and carrots, and heat in microwave for about 60 seconds. Wrap mixture in tortillas, and heat for an additional 10 to 15 seconds.

403 calories, 2 g total fat, 0 g saturated fat, 0 mg cholesterol, 405 mg sodium, 91 g carbohydrates, 19 g fiber, 20 g protein

Time Crunch

Prep once, eat twice. If you have difficulty packing a healthy lunch every day, make a larger portion of your dinner and take leftovers to lunch.

Week One Flex Dinners

Olive, Fennel, and Goat Cheese Flatbread

Flatbread pizza is a hot, new food trend. This version uses the subtle licorice flavor of fresh fennel, but get creative and top the flatbread with your own vegetable combos.

- 1 whole-grain flatbread (brand such as Flatout)
- 2 tablespoons canned sliced black olives, rinsed and drained
- ½ cup canned no-salt-added diced tomatoes, drained
- ¼ bulb fennel, thinly sliced
- 1½ ounces goat cheese, crumbled
- 3 tablespoons pine nuts
- 1½ cups low-sodium tomato soup (brands with less than 500 mg sodium per cup), heated

Preheat oven to 350°F. Bake flatbread on cookie sheet for 7 minutes. Top baked flatbread with olives, tomatoes, fennel, goat cheese, and pine nuts. Bake an additional 15 minutes. Serve with heated soup.

489 calories, 32 g total fat, 8 g saturated fat, 20 mg cholesterol, 694 mg sodium, 40 g carbohydrates, 11 g fiber, 22 g protein

Flex Swap 1½ ounces goat cheese with 1½ ounces vegetarian cheese.

Curried Quinoa Salad

This is one of the most attractive meals you will ever eat—the bright yellow of curry powder pairs well with red dried cranberries and green onion pieces. It is great by itself or topped with lean proteins such as fish or chicken.

½ cup water
¼ cup uncooked quinoa
½ teaspoon curry powder
½ cup shredded carrots
2 tablespoons dried cranberries
3 green onions, chopped
1 cup canned garbanzo beans, rinsed and drained

Bring water to a boil, and add quinoa and curry. Simmer covered for 15 minutes. Mix together carrots, cranberries, green onions, and beans. Serve carrot mixture on top of quinoa or stir all ingredients together.

510 calories, 7 g total fat, 1 g saturated fat, 0 mg cholesterol, 70 mg sodium, 95 g carbohydrates, 19 g fiber, 22 g protein

Flex Swap 1 cup garbanzo beans with a 4-ounce piece of cooked salmon, tuna, or other fish.

Edamame Stir-Fry with Brown Rice

I finally figured out the secret to a delicious homemade stir-fry: sesame oil + fresh ginger + garlic. It tastes better than takeout.

½-inch chunk ginger, grated
1 clove garlic, minced
Pinch of crushed red pepper flakes
Dash of salt
1 red bell pepper, sliced
2 teaspoons sesame oil
¾ cup shelled frozen edamame
¼ cup 100 percent pineapple juice
1 cup cooked brown rice (precooked microwavable or, if time allows, simmer your own)

Sauté the ginger, garlic, crushed red pepper, salt, and bell pepper in oil over medium heat for 3 minutes. Add edamame and pineapple juice, and cook for 8 minutes more on high heat. Heat microwavable brown rice. Top brown rice with veggie stir-fry.

485 calories, 15 g total fat, 2 g saturated fat, 0 mg cholesterol, 327 mg sodium, 74 g carbohydrates, 12 g fiber, 16 g protein

Flex Swap ¾ cup edamame for 3 ounces of cooked chicken breast or lean steak strips.

Pesto-Style Portobello Penne

Making pesto usually requires the use of a blender or food processor, but this version incorporates pesto ingredients (basil, pine nuts, olive oil, and Parmesan) without pureeing them together. A great way to save cleanup time!

- ⅔ cup (2 ounces) uncooked whole-grain penne
- 1 large portobello mushroom, sliced
- ½ cup canned cannellini beans, rinsed and drained
- 2 teaspoons olive oil
- 1 tablespoon pine nuts, toasted
- ¼ cup chopped fresh basil
- 2 tablespoons grated Parmesan

Cook pasta al dente per package directions. Sauté mushroom slices and beans in oil over medium heat for 3 to 4 minutes. Toss with all remaining ingredients.

505 calories, 19 g total fat, 4 g saturated fat, 9 mg cholesterol, 165 mg sodium, 67 g carbohydrates, 9 g fiber, 22 g protein

Flex Swap ½ cup cannellini beans for 2 ounces cooked, diced chicken breast.

Barbecue Tofu, Kale, and Sweet Potatoes

This meal is a take on hearty, Southern comfort food. Learn to love your leafy greens with this meal—the barbecue sauce and sweet potatoes tone down the natural bitter flavor of the greens.

1 cup extra-firm tofu (press to remove excess water)
1 tablespoon olive oil, split
2 tablespoons barbecue sauce, split
1 small sweet potato
2 teaspoons maple syrup
1 clove garlic, minced
3 cups chopped kale

Cut tofu into ½-inch cubes. Heat 2 teaspoons oil in skillet over medium heat. Add tofu and cook until golden, about 12 minutes (turning only two to three times). Toss warm, golden tofu with 1 tablespoon barbecue sauce. Poke the sweet potato two to three times, microwave for 10 minutes, cut in half, and top with maple syrup. In skillet sauté in remaining 1 teaspoon oil the garlic, kale, and remaining 1 tablespoon barbecue sauce until kale is tender, about 6 minutes. Serve greens with tofu on top and maple sweet potato on the side.

503 calories, 26 g total fat, 3 g saturated fat, 0 mg cholesterol, 167 mg sodium, 50 g carbohydrates, 8 g fiber, 27 g protein

Flex Swap 1 cup tofu with a 4-ounce piece of cooked salmon, tuna, or other fish.

Barley Basilico and Garlic Eggplant

I have tried preparing eggplant in many ways, and my favorite by far is ½-inch broiled slices. The slices are rolled with this basil, white bean, and barley filling.

¾ cup water
¼ cup uncooked hulled barley
1 small eggplant (with skin), sliced *lengthwise* into ½-inch pieces
Cooking spray
1 clove garlic, minced
½ cup chopped fresh basil
2 teaspoons olive oil
Dash of salt
½ cup canned Great Northern beans, rinsed and drained

Bring water to a boil. Add barley and simmer (covered) 45 minutes. Spray eggplant with cooking spray, and broil eggplant slices for 15 minutes until golden (turning once). Spread minced garlic over cooked eggplant. Stir cooked barley with basil, olive oil, salt, and beans. Put barley-and-bean mixture on short edges of cooked eggplant and roll. Optional: top with warm spaghetti sauce.

490 calories, 13 g total fat, 2 g saturated fat, 0 mg cholesterol, 337 mg sodium, 82 g carbohydrates, 28 g fiber, 19 g protein

Note: You can make the barley ahead of time in larger batches to save time. See Part Two, pages 45–46, for more barley information. Instead of barley, you can use the same amount of whole wheat couscous because it cooks in less than 15 minutes.

Lentil and Feta Bulgur with Broccoli Raab

Broccoli raab (pronounced "rob") has a more pungent, bitter taste than broccoli. If you don't buy broccoli raab, you can use broccoli. Although they are not from the same plant, they can be interchanged in recipes.

- ½ cup water
- ¼ cup uncooked bulgur
- ¾ cup canned lentils, rinsed and drained
- 1 ounce feta cheese, crumbled
- 1 lemon, juiced
- 2 tablespoons chopped fresh dill
- 1 clove garlic, minced
- 1 tablespoon olive oil
- 1½ cups chopped broccoli raab

Bring water to a boil. Add bulgur and simmer (covered) 15 minutes. Mix cooked bulgur with lentils, feta, lemon juice, and dill. Sauté garlic in oil over medium heat for 2 minutes, add broccoli raab, and cook for another 5 minutes (until tender). Serve broccoli raab on bulgur mixture.

498 calories, 21 g total fat, 6 g saturated fat, 25 mg cholesterol, 350 mg sodium, 61 g carbohydrates, 19 g fiber, 23 g protein

Flex Swap 1 ounce feta cheese with 2 tablespoons pine nuts.

Week One Flex Snacks and Desserts

Raisins and Soy Nuts

This is a quick snack. Measure it out ahead of time so you can stick to the 150-calorie portion.

1 tablespoon raisins
¼ cup soy nuts

Mix raisins and soy nuts together.

151 calories, 6 g total fat, 1 g saturated fat, 0 mg cholesterol, 39 mg sodium, 19 g carbohydrates, 5 g fiber, 9 g protein

Craving Control

Cut down on candy to perk up. According to research, people report that after they eat candy, they have reduced energy, increased tiredness, and more tension. Choose healthy snacks to energize instead.

Honey-Cinnamon Grapefruit

After you drizzle on the honey and add a dash of cinnamon, you can broil the grapefruit halves for 7 to 8 minutes to bring out more natural sweetness.

1 large grapefruit
2 teaspoons honey
Dash of cinnamon

Cut grapefruit in half and loosen segments with a knife. Drizzle honey and cinnamon on grapefruit halves.

149 calories, 0 g total fat, 0 g saturated fat, 0 mg cholesterol, 1 mg sodium, 39 g carbohydrates, 4 g fiber, 2 g protein

Green Apple and Peanut Butter Dip

I love peanut butter, but it has 100 calories in just one tablespoon. This recipe gives you the delicious peanut butter taste with only 50 calories per tablespoon and some soybean nutrition! It is great for spreading or for dipping other fruits and vegetables, such as carrots, celery, and red peppers.

2 tablespoons Peanut Butter Dip (see following recipe)
1 small green apple, sliced

Make Peanut Butter Dip. Spread on apple slices.

155 calories, 8 g total fat, 2 g saturated fat, 0 mg cholesterol, 16 mg sodium, 18 g carbohydrates, 4 g fiber, 5 g protein

Peanut Butter Dip

Makes 8 servings (2 tablespoons each)

⅓ container (½ cup) silken tofu (lite, firm)
½ cup natural peanut butter

Puree tofu with hand blender until completely smooth. Blend in peanut butter. Keep covered in fridge for 5 to 7 days.

Protein Popcorn

My girlfriend Kris convinced me to eat nutritional yeast sprinkled on popcorn. Nutritional yeast tastes like Parmesan cheese but has far more nutrition. Two tablespoons of nutritional yeast has four times more fiber and double the protein of Parmesan, plus it is packed with the B vitamins that vegetarians need! Give it a shake.

- 2 tablespoons popcorn (or 1 100-calorie minibag of microwave popcorn)
- Cooking spray
- 2 tablespoons nutritional yeast

Pop the corn, spray with cooking spray, and sprinkle with nutritional yeast.

153 calories, 2 g total fat, 0 g saturated fat, 0 mg cholesterol, 11 mg sodium, 28 g carbohydrates, 9 g fiber, 10 g protein

Note: For the most natural popcorn, put popcorn kernels in a plain brown lunch bag and fold the open end over three to four times tightly. Microwave for about 2 to 3 minutes (until pops are about 5 seconds apart).

Maple Yogurt

This is so delicious that my grandma thought it was decadent whipped cream!

1 container (6 ounces) low-fat, plain, Greek-style yogurt (such as Fage or Stonyfield Oikos)
1 tablespoon 100 percent maple syrup

Mix yogurt with maple syrup.

153 calories, 3 g total fat, 2 g saturated fat, 10 mg cholesterol, 113 mg sodium, 25 g carbohydrates, 0 g fiber, 8 g protein

Craving Control

Keep a "munch log" to help control oversnacking. Instead of keeping a food log of your entire day, just write down what you snack on between meals. This keeps you mindful of munchies.

Broiled Banana with Walnuts

Broiled bananas develop a delicate caramel flavor and creamy texture. Broil and serve in the banana skin for an impressive presentation.

1 medium banana
1 tablespoon chopped walnuts

Cut banana lengthwise, leaving the peel on. Place on baking sheet, and broil flesh side up for about 5 to 6 minutes until banana is golden or caramelized. Sprinkle walnuts on top. Serve in banana peel.

154 calories, 5 g total fat, 1 g saturated fat, 0 mg cholesterol, 1 mg sodium, 28 g carbohydrates, 4 g fiber, 2 g protein

Apple and Cranberry Skillet Crisp

The chewy cranberries and toasted oats on top elevate chopped apples to true decadence.

- 3 tablespoons raw old-fashioned or rolled oats
- 1 small apple, chopped
- 1 tablespoon dried cranberries
- 1 teaspoon maple syrup
- 2 tablespoons water

In dry skillet over medium heat, toss raw oatmeal until golden, about 4 minutes, and set aside. In same skillet, put chopped apple, cranberries, maple syrup, and water. Simmer on low (covered) for 5 to 6 minutes, until apple is tender. Top with oats.

152 calories, 1 g total fat, 0 g saturated fat, 0 mg cholesterol, 3 mg sodium, 35 g carbohydrates, 4 g fiber, 3 g protein

Week One Flex Shopping List

Make sure you have your fridge, pantry, and spice rack staples stocked (pages 79–80). Amounts in parentheses indicate how much you will use this week.

This list is for one person; multiply the ingredients if you are cooking for more. Check off what you need from the grocery store this week.

Grains

- ☐ Bagel, whole grain (1)
- ☐ Barley, hulled (¼ cup uncooked)
- ☐ Bread, whole grain (1 slice)
- ☐ Brown rice (about 2 cups precooked microwavable or ⅔ cup uncooked)
- ☐ Bulgur (¼ cup uncooked)
- ☐ Crunchy granola bar, whole grain (1)
- ☐ Flatbread, whole grain (1)
- ☐ Hamburger bun, whole grain (1)
- ☐ Oats, rolled (1¼ cups)
- ☐ Penne, whole grain (⅔ cup uncooked = 2 ounces uncooked)
- ☐ Pita pocket, whole grain (1)
- ☐ Popcorn (1 microwavable 100-calorie minibag or 2 tablespoons popcorn)
- ☐ Quinoa (¼ cup uncooked)
- ☐ Tortillas, whole grain (6 small)

Fruit

- ☐ 100 percent pineapple juice (¼ cup)
- ☐ Apples (4)
- ☐ Apricots, dried (3)
- ☐ Avocado (1)
- ☐ Bananas (2)
- ☐ Cranberries, dried (3 tablespoons)
- ☐ Figs, dried (2)
- ☐ Grapefruit (1)
- ☐ Orange (1)
- ☐ Raisins (3 tablespoons)
- ☐ Red grapes (½ cup)

Fresh Herbs and Flavorings

- ☐ Basil, fresh (about 1 cup)
- ☐ Chives, fresh (1 tablespoon)
- ☐ Dill, fresh (2 tablespoons)
- ☐ Ginger, fresh (½-inch chunk)
- ☐ Parsley, fresh (1 tablespoon)

Vegetables

- ☐ Bell pepper, red (1)
- ☐ Broccoli raab (1½ cups)
- ☐ Carrots, shredded (1¼ cups)
- ☐ Cherry tomatoes (1½ cups)
- ☐ Eggplant (1 small)
- ☐ Fennel bulb (¼)
- ☐ Green onions (3)
- ☐ Green spring salad mix (6 cups salad)
- ☐ Kale (3 cups)
- ☐ Portobello mushroom (1 large)
- ☐ Potato (½ small)
- ☐ Romaine lettuce (1 cup)
- ☐ Sweet potato (1 small)
- ☐ Tomato (1 medium)

Nuts, Seeds, and Miscellaneous

- ☐ Almonds (3 tablespoons, sliced)
- ☐ Flaxseed, ground (1 tablespoon)
- ☐ Nutritional yeast (2 tablespoons)
- ☐ Pecans (1 tablespoon, chopped)
- ☐ Pine nuts (5 tablespoons)
- ☐ Soy nuts (¼ cup)
- ☐ Walnuts (5 tablespoons, chopped)

Refrigerated Products

- ☐ Cheddar cheese (2 slices)
- ☐ Cottage cheese, low fat (½ cup)
- ☐ Eggs (1 whole + 2 whites)
- ☐ Feta cheese (1 ounce)

- ☐ Goat cheese (1½ ounces)
- ☐ Greek-style plain yogurt, low fat (6-ounce container)
- ☐ Mozzarella cheese, fresh (1 ounce)
- ☐ Parmesan cheese (2 tablespoons, grated)
- ☐ Plain yogurt, low fat (6-ounce container)
- ☐ Tofu, extra firm (1 cup)
- ☐ Silken tofu, lite, firm (½ cup)

Canned and Frozen Goods

- ☐ Artichoke hearts, canned in water (3 hearts)
- ☐ Black beans, canned (¾ cup)
- ☐ Black olives, canned and sliced (2 tablespoons)
- ☐ Cannellini beans, canned (1¼ cups)
- ☐ Garbanzo beans, canned (1 cup)
- ☐ Great Northern beans, canned (½ cup)
- ☐ Lentils, canned (1½ cups)
- ☐ Refried beans, canned low-fat or vegetarian (¾ cup)
- ☐ Frozen edamame, or shelled green soybeans (1 cup)
- ☐ Frozen mixed berries, unsweetened (1 cup)
- ☐ Frozen waffles, whole grain (2)
- ☐ Low-sodium tomato soup (1½ cups)
- ☐ Vegetarian sausage-style crumbles (¼ cup)
- ☐ Veggie burger (1)

Week Two Recipes, Meal Plan, Shopping List

Week Two Flex Breakfasts

Fruit and Nut Polenta

Polenta is not usually considered for a morning cereal, but it is a nice change of pace. This version is made with 50 percent water and 50 percent milk for added creaminess.

- ½ cup water
- ½ cup skim milk or soy milk
- ¼ cup polenta (medium-grind whole-grain cornmeal)
- ¼ cup frozen unsweetened cherries, thawed and chopped
- 2 tablespoons chopped hazelnuts
- 2 teaspoons agave nectar

Bring water and milk to a boil, and slowly sprinkle in polenta while whisking. Simmer and stir for about 15 minutes (until water is absorbed). Take off from heat, and top with cherries, nuts, and agave nectar.

303 calories, 10 g total fat, 1 g saturated fat, 2 mg cholesterol, 67 mg sodium, 48 g carbohydrates, 4 g fiber, 9 g protein

Vanilla-Date Oatmeal

Dates are naturally high in sugar, so they add delicious chewy sweetness. The hint of vanilla also lends a mild, sweet flavor, and if you are in the mood to splurge, use a bit of vanilla bean (about four to five dollars each) instead of the extract.

1 cup skim milk or soy milk
½ cup rolled oats
2 dates, chopped
½ teaspoon vanilla extract
1 teaspoon honey

Bring milk and oats to a boil. Simmer and stir for 5 minutes. Add dates, vanilla, and honey.

310 calories, 3 g total fat, 1 g saturated fat, 5 mg cholesterol, 105 mg sodium, 57 g carbohydrates, 5 g fiber, 15 g protein

Cranberry and Walnut Barley with Honey

The hearty chewy texture of barley is a nice morning alternative to oatmeal. As most people don't have the time to wait around for barley to cook in the morning, make a big batch ahead of time keep it in the fridge and warm in the microwave for a healthy breakfast in a hurry all week.

- ¾ cup water
- ¼ cup uncooked hulled barley
- 1 tablespoon dried cranberries
- 2 tablespoons chopped walnuts
- 1 teaspoon honey

Bring water to a boil. Add barley and simmer (covered) 45 minutes. Stir in cranberries, walnuts, and honey.

303 calories, 11 g total fat, 1 g saturated fat, 0 mg cholesterol, 12 mg sodium, 47 g carbohydrates, 9 g fiber, 8 g protein

Note: You can make barley ahead of time in larger batches to save time. You can also substitute ½ cup rolled oats for the barley because it will take only 5 minutes cooking time.

Florentine-Scramble Breakfast Sandwich

This spinach-omelet breakfast sandwich is a delicious way to eat leafy greens early in the day.

Cooking spray
1 cup baby spinach
1 egg, beaten
Dash of black pepper
1 vegetarian sausage patty, heated
1 whole-grain English muffin, toasted

Spray pan with cooking spray, and sauté spinach for 1 minute until wilted. In same pan, scramble egg with spinach and black pepper. Put scrambled eggs and hot vegetarian sausage patty on English muffin.

311 calories, 14 g total fat, 3 g saturated fat, 212 mg cholesterol, 603 mg sodium, 32 g carbohydrates, 7 g fiber, 20 g protein

Flex Swap 1 vegetarian sausage patty with 2 ounces uncured Canadian bacon.

Peanut-Butter-Banana Smoothie

The peanut butter and banana make this a really thick shake that sticks with you.

1 cup (8 ounces) low-fat plain kefir (drinkable yogurt product)
1 tablespoon peanut butter
1 small banana

Blend kefir, peanut butter, and banana with hand blender until smooth. Add ice cubes for even thicker consistency.

298 calories, 11 g total fat, 3 g saturated fat, 9 mg cholesterol, 332 mg sodium, 42 g carbohydrates, 4 g fiber, 13 g protein

Feeling Good

Take a cigarette-free smoke break. It's not healthy to smoke, but it is healthy to go outside for a puff of fresh air. When you feel office boredom, procrastination, or fatigue, go outside for a few minutes to get refreshed instead of visiting a candy dish or vending machine.

Apple and Almond Butter Toast

I used to eat peanut butter on toast with sliced apples—until I bought my first jar of almond butter. Now I am hooked on it.

- 1 slice whole-grain bread, toasted
- 1½ tablespoons almond butter
- 1 small apple, sliced

Spread almond butter on toast. Top with apple slices.

295 calories, 15 g total fat, 2 g saturated fat, 0 mg cholesterol, 142 mg sodium, 37 g carbohydrates, 6 g fiber, 7 g protein

Waffles with Figgie-Pear Sauce

Figgie-pear sauce adds a sweet kick to healthy whole-grain waffles. The sauce can also be used on top of yogurt or oatmeal.

½ pear, diced
2 dried figs, diced
1 teaspoon maple syrup
Dash of vanilla extract
2 frozen whole-grain waffles, toasted

In a covered pot over medium heat, simmer pear, figs, maple syrup, and vanilla for 5 minutes, until pear is mushy. Top toasted waffles with figgie-pear sauce.

308 calories, 9 g total fat, 2 g saturated fat, 0 mg cholesterol, 332 mg sodium, 54 g carbohydrates, 6 g fiber, 7 g protein

Week Two Flex Lunches

Marinated Garden Lentil Pita

Ordinary ingredients come together to make an extraordinary fast and fresh meal.

- ¾ cup canned lentils, rinsed and drained
- ½ cup chopped cucumber
- ½ cup shredded carrots
- ½ red bell pepper, chopped
- 2 tablespoons Universal Lemon-Flax Vinaigrette (see Index) or low-fat Italian dressing
- 1 whole-grain pita pocket, cut in half

Mix lentils, cucumber, carrots, and bell pepper with vinaigrette. Stuff mixture into pita halves.

410 calories, 11 g total fat, 1 g saturated fat, 0 mg cholesterol, 279 mg sodium, 65 g carbohydrates, 19 g fiber, 19 g protein

BLT (Balsamic, Lettuce, and Tomato)

Balsamic vinegar drizzled on thick slices of red tomatoes is simple but tastes gourmet. If your tomatoes aren't flavorful, cut them in half, and broil them flesh side up for 5 minutes to bring out natural flavors. You could also use roasted red peppers packed in water in place of the tomatoes.

4 tablespoons hummus
2 slices whole-grain bread, toasted
¼ avocado, mashed
2 pieces of romaine lettuce
2 thick slices of tomato
1 tablespoon balsamic vinegar
½ cup grapes

Spread hummus on one slice of toast and avocado on the other. Top hummus side with lettuce and tomato, and drizzle with vinegar. Close sandwich. Serve with grapes.

410 calories, 15 g total fat, 2 g saturated fat, 0 mg cholesterol, 434 mg sodium, 62 g carbohydrates, 11 g fiber, 11 g protein

Black Bean and Zucchini Quesadillas

The microwave makes the tortillas warm and tender, but if you like your quesadillas with a little crunch, use the broiler or toaster oven.

½ cup chopped zucchini
½ cup canned black beans, rinsed and drained
2 green onions, chopped
½ teaspoon cumin
¼ teaspoon chili powder
1 lime, juiced
2 small (6-inch) whole-grain tortillas
1-ounce slice cheddar cheese, cut in half

In bowl, mix zucchini, beans, onions, cumin, chili powder, and lime juice together. Fill each tortilla with zucchini and bean mixture, top with a half-slice of cheese, and heat in microwave for 60 seconds. Fold in half.

409 calories, 11 g total fat, 6 g saturated fat, 29 mg cholesterol, 537 mg sodium, 70 g carbohydrates, 13 g fiber, 22 g protein

Flex Swap 1 slice cheddar cheese with ¼ avocado, diced, or 1 slice of vegetarian cheese.

Barbecue Baja Burger

Avocado and barbecue sauce together make this burger fresh tasting, sweet, and smoky.

1 vegetarian burger
1 whole-grain hamburger bun
¼ avocado, sliced
¼ cup sprouts (broccoli, radish, or alfalfa)
2 tablespoons barbecue sauce
1 orange

Heat burger in microwave, place on bun, and top with avocado, sprouts, and barbecue sauce. Serve with an orange.

410 calories, 15 g total fat, 2 g saturated fat, 0 mg cholesterol, 637 mg sodium, 55 g carbohydrates, 14 g fiber, 19 g protein

Flex Swap veggie burger for 3 ounces sliced turkey breast or 3 ounces cooked extra-lean turkey or beef burger.

Sunflower Seed Salad

After creating this recipe, I immediately e-mailed my girlfriends to try it. Sunflower seeds, green apples, green onions, and red peppers mingle so flavorfully together.

1 tablespoon sunflower seed butter
1 tablespoon warm water
2 tablespoons white balsamic vinegar
Dash of crushed red pepper flakes
¾ cup canned garbanzo beans, rinsed and drained
½ apple, diced
3 green onions, diced
½ red bell pepper, diced
3 cups green spring salad mix

Mix sunflower seed butter, water, vinegar, and crushed red pepper together. Toss together with remaining salad ingredients.

389 calories, 11 g total fat, 1 g saturated fat, 0 mg cholesterol, 65 mg sodium, 60 g carbohydrates, 16 g fiber, 18 g protein

Flex Swap ¾ cup garbanzo beans for 3 ounces cooked, diced chicken breast.

Spicy Beans and Greens Burrito

Green chilies gained a special place in my heart after I lived in New Mexico, where they are found in almost every breakfast, lunch, and dinner meal. They give the green spinach and beans a spicy kick without being overpowering.

- ¾ cup low-fat or vegetarian refried beans
- 3 tablespoons canned diced green chilies
- 2 small (6-inch) whole-grain tortillas
- 1½ cups baby spinach
- 1-ounce slice cheddar cheese, cut in half

In bowl, stir beans with green chilies, and heat in microwave for 60 to 90 seconds. Spread hot beans on tortillas, and top with spinach and cheese.

411 calories, 11 g total fat, 6 g saturated fat, 28 mg cholesterol, 713 mg sodium, 68 g carbohydrates, 11 g fiber, 23 g protein

Flex Swap 1 ounce sliced cheddar cheese with 1 slice vegetarian cheese.

Arugula Salad with Fig and Goat Cheese

The sweet fig and goat cheese tone down arugula's naturally bitter and peppery flavor.

3 cups arugula
3 dried figs, chopped
1 ounce goat cheese, crumbled
2 tablespoons balsamic vinegar
½ cup canned Great Northern beans, rinsed and drained
2 tablespoons chopped walnuts

Toss all ingredients together.

404 calories, 17 g total fat, 5 g saturated fat, 13 mg cholesterol, 136 mg sodium, 48 g carbohydrates, 10 g fiber, 19 g protein

Flex Swap ½ cup Great Northern beans for 2 ounces cooked, diced chicken breast.

Week Two Flex Dinners

Black Bean Taco Salad

The lime, garlic, and cumin salad dressing can also be used to marinate fish or chicken. This salad is tossed with just enough crushed chips to offer a nice texture contrast to the creamy avocado and tender black beans.

1 lime, juiced
1 tablespoon olive oil
1 teaspoon cumin
1 clove garlic, minced
Dash of salt
¾ cup canned black beans, rinsed and drained
3 cups shredded romaine lettuce
1 tomato, chopped
10 whole-grain tortilla chips, crushed
¼ avocado, chopped

Whisk together lime juice, oil, cumin, garlic, and salt. Toss all ingredients together.

495 calories, 27 g total fat, 4 g saturated fat, 0 mg cholesterol, 186 mg sodium, 56 g carbohydrates, 15 g fiber, 15 g protein

Flex Swap ½ cup black beans for 2 ounces cooked, diced chicken breast.

Pad-Thai-Style Tempeh

The flavor combination of sour lime plus salty peanuts equals a truly pleasurable taste-bud experience.

2 ounces (dime's circumference) whole-grain fettuccine, uncooked
2 teaspoons peanut oil
1 lime, juiced
1 clove garlic, minced
Dash of salt
2 ounces (¼ of 8-ounce package) tempeh, cut in ½-inch cubes
1½ cups broccoli coleslaw (Mann's brand)
1 tablespoon chopped peanuts
2 green onions, chopped

Cook pasta al dente per package directions. Sauté oil, lime juice, garlic, salt, and tempeh cubes for about 5 minutes. Add coleslaw, and cook for another 3 minutes. Toss cooked pasta with tempeh mixture. Top with peanuts and green onions.

499 calories, 20 g total fat, 4 g saturated fat, 0 mg cholesterol, 209 mg sodium, 64 g carbohydrates, 6 g fiber, 25 g protein

Flex Swap 2 ounces of tempeh for 2 ounces (9 medium) frozen cooked shrimp, thawed.

Zucchini Fritters with Green Salad

These fritters meet strict comfort-food guidelines—crunchy outside, warm and tender inside.

¾ cup canned Great Northern beans, rinsed and drained
1 zucchini, grated
¼ cup grated onion
¼ cup whole wheat flour
1 tablespoon Italian seasoning
Dash of salt and black pepper
1 teaspoon olive oil
2 cups green spring salad mix
2 tablespoons Universal Lemon-Flax Vinaigrette (see Index) or low-fat Italian dressing

With hand blender, puree beans. Stir in zucchini, onion, flour, Italian seasoning, salt, and black pepper. Form four patties. In a nonstick skillet over medium heat with 1 teaspoon oil, brown fritters 4 minutes on each side. Toss salad with vinaigrette. Serve fritters on salad.

487 calories, 16 g total fat, 2 g saturated fat, 0 mg cholesterol, 272 mg sodium, 73 g carbohydrates, 22 g fiber, 20 g protein

Sage-Mushroom Barley with Parmesan

The many savory (umami) ingredients, such as mushrooms, Parmesan, and sage, make this a meaty-flavored vegetarian dish.

- ¾ cup water
- ¼ cup uncooked hulled barley
- 1 cup sliced fresh mushrooms
- ½ onion, chopped
- 1 clove garlic, minced
- 1 teaspoon dried sage
- 2 teaspooons olive oil
- ½ cup canned navy beans, rinsed and drained
- 1 cup chopped fresh baby spinach
- 2 tablespoons grated Parmesan cheese

Bring water to a boil. Add barley and simmer (covered) 45 minutes. Sauté mushrooms, onions, garlic, and sage in oil over medium heat for 4 to 5 minutes, until mushrooms are tender. Add beans and cook for 1 to 2 minutes. Take off from heat, and toss mixture with spinach and cooked barley. Top with Parmesan.

488 calories, 14 g total fat, 3 g saturated fat, 9 mg cholesterol, 207 mg sodium, 73 g carbohydrates, 16 g fiber, 23 g protein

Note: You can make barley ahead of time in larger batches to save time. See Part Two, pages 45–46, for more barley information. You can substitute 2 ounces of whole-grain pasta for the barley because the pasta has a shorter cooking time.

Tortilla and Cheddar Chili

Chili can be a fast meal fix, but adding a bit of crunchy chips and gooey cheese makes it a meal to remember.

- ¼ onion, diced
- 1 green bell pepper, diced
- 1 jalapeño pepper, diced without veins or seeds
- 1 clove garlic, minced
- 2 tablespoons chili powder
- 2 teaspoons olive oil
- 1 cup canned no-salt-added *crushed* tomatoes (*not* drained)
- ½ cup canned kidney beans, rinsed and drained
- 1 cup water
- ½ slice cheddar cheese, chopped into pieces, or ½ ounce cheddar cheese, shredded
- 10 whole-grain tortillas chips, crushed

Sauté onion, green pepper, jalapeño, garlic, and chili powder in oil over medium heat for 5 minutes, until pepper is tender. Add tomatoes, beans, and water, and bring to a boil. Remove from heat, and top with cheese and tortillas.

490 calories, 22 g total fat, 5 g saturated fat, 15 mg cholesterol, 292 mg sodium, 64 g carbohydrates, 20 g fiber, 19 g protein

Flex Swap ½ ounce cheddar chesse with ½ ounce vegetarian cheese.

Polenta Pizza Bake

This is a quick pizza casserole that uses cornmeal (polenta) as the crust. Cornmeal crusts can be found at many classic Chicago pizzerias.

- 2 cups water
- ½ cup polenta (medium-grind whole-grain cornmeal)
- Dash of salt and black pepper
- Cooking spray
- 1 clove garlic, minced
- 1 tablespoon Italian seasoning
- ½ cup vegetarian sausage-style crumbles (in frozen or produce department)
- 2 teaspoons olive oil
- 1 cup canned no-salt-added *crushed* tomatoes (*not* drained)
- 1 tablespoon balsamic vinegar
- 2 tablespoons grated part-skim mozzarella cheese

Bring water to a boil, and slowly sprinkle in polenta, salt, and black pepper while whisking. Simmer and stir for about 15 minutes (until water is absorbed). Spray an 8-inch casserole dish with cooking spray; then spread polenta evenly on the bottom. Sauté garlic, Italian seasoning, and vegetarian crumbles in oil for 3 minutes. Stir in tomatoes and vinegar, and bring to boil. Spoon tomato mixture on polenta, and top with cheese. Broil until cheese is golden.

504 calories, 17 g total fat, 4 g saturated fat, 8 mg cholesterol, 530 mg sodium, 68 g carbohydrates, 11 g fiber, 22 g protein

Flex Swap ½ cup vegetarian crumbles for 2 ounces cooked *extra-lean* ground turkey or sirloin.

Roasted Tomato and White Bean Penne

The colors and flavors will have you thinking you are in Italy—fresh green basil, red tomatoes, and white beans are the colors of Italy's flag.

⅔ cup (2 ounces) uncooked whole-grain penne
1 cup cherry tomatoes, whole
3 cloves garlic, whole
1 tablespoon olive oil, split
Dash of salt and black pepper
½ cup canned cannellini beans, rinsed and drained
¼ cup chopped fresh basil
1 tablespoon grated Parmesan cheese

Cook pasta al dente per package directions (reserve 4 tablespoons of cooking water). Toss whole tomatoes and whole garlic cloves with 1 teaspoon oil, salt, and black pepper. Place on cookie sheet, and broil for 8 minutes until tomatoes start bursting and garlic is tender. Mash broiled garlic with remaining 2 teaspoons olive oil and 4 tablespoons cooking water from the pasta. Toss all ingredients together.

511 calories, 17 g total fat, 3 g saturated fat, 4 mg cholesterol, 257 mg sodium, 76 g carbohydrates, 13 g fiber, 21 g protein

Week Two Flex Snacks and Desserts

Pizza Popcorn

It always surprises people that this tastes just like pizza!

- 2 tablespoons popcorn (or 100-calorie minibag of microwave popcorn)
- Cooking spray
- 2 tablespoons Italian seasoning
- 2 tablespoons grated Parmesan cheese

Pop the corn, spray with cooking spray, and sprinkle with Italian seasoning and cheese.

161 calories, 4 g total fat, 2 g saturated fat, 9 mg cholesterol, 156 mg sodium, 24 g carbohydrates, 5 g fiber, 8 g protein

Note: For the most natural popcorn, put the popcorn kernels in a plain brown lunch bag and fold the open end over three to four times tightly. Microwave for about 2 to 3 minutes (until pops are about 5 seconds apart).

Flex Swap 2 tablespoons Parmesan cheese with 2 tablespoons nutritional yeast.

Pistachios

Keep a stash in your purse, glove compartment, and desk to stave off hunger when it strikes. Premeasure the portions so you can stick to the 1-ounce portion, and be sure to get them in-the-shell to help you slow down and savor the flavor. This is my favorite snack.

50 pistachios (1 ounce) in shell

158 calories, 13 g total fat, 2 g saturated fat, 0 mg cholesterol, 0 mg sodium, 8 g carbohydrates, 3 g fiber, 6 g protein

Apple and Cheddar

This is a sweet and savory snack combination.

1 small apple, sliced
1-ounce slice cheddar cheese

157 calories, 9 g total fat, 5 g saturated fat, 26 mg cholesterol, 158 mg sodium, 15 g carbohydrates, 3 g fiber, 7 g protein

Flex Swap 1 slice cheddar cheese with 1 slice vegetarian cheddar cheese.

Hummus and Jicama

Jicama is a beautiful white, crunchy vegetable that hides under a brown, unattractive outer peel. It also tastes great sliced with a squeeze of lime.

¼ cup hummus
1 cup jicama slices

Dip jicama slices into hummus.

152 calories, 5 total g fat, 1 g saturated fat, 0 mg cholesterol, 150 mg sodium, 23 g carbohydrates, 8 g fiber, 4 g protein

Mexican Hot Chocolate

Who knew that cinnamon and honey taste so good with chocolate? Cinnamon has a naturally sugar-free sweet taste, so you can get away with using only a small amount of honey.

1 cup (8 ounces) skim milk or soy milk
1 tablespoon unsweetened cocoa powder
1 tablespoon honey
Dash of cinnamon

In a saucepan, bring milk to almost a boil. In a mug, stir cocoa, honey, and cinnamon together, and *slowly* add hot milk into cocoa mixture, stirring until smooth.

160 calories, 1 g total fat, 1 g saturated fat, 5 mg cholesterol, 105 mg sodium, 33 g carbohydrates, 2 g fiber, 9 g protein

Cinnamon-Spice Peaches with Pecans

Broiling or grilling peaches with just a few dashes of spice makes them more special and sweet than eating them raw.

1 peach, cut in half and pit removed
1 teaspoon pie spice (apple or pumpkin)
4 teaspoons chopped pecans, toasted
2 teaspoons agave nectar

Broil peach halves flesh side up for 6 to 8 minutes, until tender. Sprinkle on spice and pecans, and drizzle with agave nectar.

149 calories, 7 g total fat, 1 g saturated fat, 0 mg cholesterol, 1 mg sodium, 23 g carbohydrates, 3 g fiber, 2 g protein

Note: You can also grill peaches on an indoor grill pan or outdoor grill. Spray a little cooking spray on the flesh, and place halves flesh side down for 6 to 8 minutes.

Chocolate Mousse with Raspberries

You won't believe this is tofu, and you won't want any other pudding or mousse after you try this. Seriously.

- 1 package (12 ounces) *silken* tofu (lite, firm)
- 2 tablespoons unsweetened cocoa powder
- 2 tablespoons agave nectar
- Dash of vanilla extract
- ½ cup raspberries

With a hand blender, puree tofu, cocoa powder, agave, and vanilla until smooth. Serve with raspberries on top.

151 calories, 2 g total fat, 1 g saturated fat, 0 mg cholesterol, 144 mg sodium, 24 g carbohydrates, 4 g fiber, 12 g protein

Note: You can make four servings at once and keep the leftovers for 3 to 4 days in the fridge—better yet, share with friends.

Week Two Flex Shopping List

Make sure you have your fridge, pantry, and spice rack staples stocked (pages 79–80). Amounts in parentheses indicate how much you will use this week.

This list is for one person; multiply the ingredients if you are cooking for more. Check off what you need from the grocery store this week.

Grains

- ☐ Barley, hulled (½ cup uncooked)
- ☐ Bread, whole grain (3 slices)
- ☐ English muffin, whole grain (1)
- ☐ Fettuccine, whole grain (2 ounces)
- ☐ Flour, whole wheat (¼ cup)
- ☐ Hamburger bun, whole grain (1)
- ☐ Oats, rolled (½ cup)
- ☐ Penne, whole grain (⅔ cup uncooked = 2 ounces uncooked)
- ☐ Pita pocket, whole grain (1)
- ☐ Polenta, medium-grind whole-grain cornmeal (¾ cup)
- ☐ Popcorn (1 microwavable 100-calorie minibag or 2 tablespoons popcorn)
- ☐ Tortillas, whole grain (4 small)

Fruit

- ☐ Apples (3)
- ☐ Avocado (1)
- ☐ Banana (1)
- ☐ Cranberries, dried (1 tablespoon)
- ☐ Dates (2)
- ☐ Figs, dried (5)
- ☐ Grapes (½ cup)
- ☐ Orange (1)
- ☐ Peach (1)
- ☐ Pear (1)
- ☐ Raspberries (½ cup)

Fresh Herbs and Flavorings

- ☐ Basil, fresh (¼ cup)

Vegetables

- ☐ Arugula (3 cups)
- ☐ Baby spinach (3½ cups)
- ☐ Bell pepper, green (1)
- ☐ Bell pepper, red (1)
- ☐ Broccoli coleslaw (1½ cups)
- ☐ Carrots, shredded (½ cup)
- ☐ Cherry tomatoes (1 cup)
- ☐ Cucumber (½ cup, sliced)
- ☐ Green onions (7)
- ☐ Green spring salad mix (5 cups)
- ☐ Jalapeño pepper (1)
- ☐ Jicama (1 cup, sliced)
- ☐ Mushrooms, sliced (1 cup)
- ☐ Romaine lettuce (about 3 cups)
- ☐ Sprouts (¼ cup)
- ☐ Tomatoes (2)
- ☐ Zucchini (2)

Nuts, Seeds, and Miscellaneous

- ☐ Agave nectar (2 tablespoons + 4 teaspoons)
- ☐ Cocoa powder, unsweetened (1 tablespoon)
- ☐ Hazelnuts (2 tablespoons, chopped)
- ☐ Peanuts (1 tablespoon, chopped)
- ☐ Pecans (4 teaspoons, chopped)
- ☐ Pistachios (50 in shell)
- ☐ Tortilla chips, whole grain (20 chips)
- ☐ Walnuts (4 tablespoons, chopped)

Refrigerated Products

- ☐ Cheddar cheese (3½ slices)
- ☐ Egg (1 whole)
- ☐ Goat cheese (1 ounce)
- ☐ Hummus (½ cup)
- ☐ Mozzarella cheese, part-skim (2 tablespoons, shredded)
- ☐ Parmesan cheese (5 tablespoons, grated)
- ☐ Plain kefir, low fat (1 cup)

- ☐ Silken tofu, lite, firm (12 ounces)
- ☐ Tempeh (2 ounces of 8-ounce package)

Canned and Frozen Goods

- ☐ Black beans, canned (1¼ cups)
- ☐ Cannellini beans, canned (½ cup)
- ☐ Garbanzo beans, canned (¾ cup)
- ☐ Great Northern beans, canned (1¼ cups)
- ☐ Green chilies, canned and diced (3 tablespoons)
- ☐ Kidney beans, canned (½ cup)
- ☐ Lentils, canned (¾ cup)
- ☐ Navy beans, canned (½ cup)
- ☐ Refried beans, canned low-fat or vegetarian (¾ cup)
- ☐ Frozen cherries, unsweetened (¼ cup)
- ☐ Frozen waffles, whole grain (2)
- ☐ Vegetarian sausage patty (1)
- ☐ Vegetarian sausage-style crumbles (½ cup)
- ☐ Veggie burger (1)

Week Three Recipes, Meal Plan, Shopping List

Week Three Flex Breakfasts

Sunflower-Raisin Oatmeal

Stirring sunflower seed butter into oatmeal makes it even creamier. Try to get a raisin in each bite, because the combo is perfect.

1 cup water
½ cup rolled oats
1 tablespoon sunflower seed butter
2 tablespoons raisins

Bring water and oats to a boil. Simmer and stir for 5 minutes. Stir in sunflower seed butter. Top with raisins.

310 calories, 10 g total fat, 1 g saturated fat, 0 mg cholesterol, 11 mg sodium, 48 g carbohydrates, 5 g fiber, 10 g protein

Banana-Nut Oatmeal

Try this for less saturated fat, double the fiber, and about 150 fewer calories than a banana-nut muffin (which can have at least 400 to 500 calories).

½ cup water
½ cup skim milk or soy milk
½ cup rolled oats
½ banana, chopped
1 tablespoon chopped walnuts

Bring water, milk, and oats to a boil. Simmer and stir for 5 minutes. Top with banana and nuts or stir it all together.

299 calories, 8 g total fat, 1 g saturated fat, 2 mg cholesterol, 57 mg sodium, 48 g carbohydrates, 6 g fiber, 12 g protein

Apple-Cranberry Bulgur Breakfast

Because bulgur is tiny, the apple and cranberries add the right amount of bite and texture to make this a hearty breakfast.

- ¼ cup water
- ¼ cup 100 percent apple juice
- ¼ cup uncooked bulgur
- ½ apple, chopped
- 2 tablespoons dried cranberries
- ½ cup (4 ounces) plain low-fat yogurt

Bring water and apple juice to a boil. Add bulgur and simmer (covered) 15 minutes. Stir bulgur with apples and cranberries, and top with yogurt.

304 calories, 3 g total fat, 1 g saturated fat, 7 mg cholesterol, 96 mg sodium, 63 g carbohydrates, 9 g fiber, 11 g protein

Swiss Broccoli Frittata with Dill

Frittatas are a one-skillet meal for a fast breakfast, brunch, or dinner option with very little cleanup. I make frittatas with about three times more vegetables than egg. For a fun presentation, put the warm and browned frittata on a cutting board and use a pizza cutter to cut it into pie-shaped wedges.

1 whole egg + 3 egg whites
1 cup finely chopped broccoli
1 slice (1 ounce) Swiss cheese, chopped into pieces
2 tablespoons chopped fresh dill
Cooking spray
¾ cup sliced strawberries

Beat egg and egg whites, and mix in broccoli, cheese, and dill. Pour into skillet sprayed with cooking spray, and cook (without stirring) for 3 to 4 minutes, until firm on bottom but slightly wet on top. Preheat oven to broil setting and broil for 3 minutes, until eggs are cooked and golden. Serve with strawberries on the side.

300 calories, 14 g total fat, 7 g saturated fat, 237 mg cholesterol, 319 mg sodium, 18 g carbohydrates, 5 g fiber, 28 g protein

Three-Cup Quickie

Cold cereal is a standard quick start to the morning. The perfect cereal equation is 1 cup whole-grain cereal + 1 cup cut fruit + 1 cup of skim or soy milk.

1 cup cold whole-grain cereal
1 cup skim milk or soy milk
1 cup blueberries

301 calories, 1 g total fat, 0 g saturated fat, 5 mg cholesterol, 357 mg sodium, 64 g carbohydrates, 7 g fiber, 12 g protein

Out and About

Know before you go. Check restaurant menus online, or call them to fax or e-mail you a copy. Make your order selections *before* you get to the restaurant, as you will have more time to think through your dining decisions.

Vanilla-Spice French Toast with Berry Syrup

Instead of fake high-fructose pancake syrups, use fresh berries warmed and mashed. You can use this fresh-fruit syrup on top of pancakes, yogurt, or ice cream, too.

1 egg + 2 egg whites
1 teaspoon vanilla extract
1 teaspoon pie spice (apple or pumpkin)
2 slices whole-grain bread
Cooking spray
⅓ cup unsweetened frozen mixed berries

Mix egg, vanilla, and spice. Lightly dip bread into egg mixture. Cook in pan sprayed with cooking spray for 3 minutes on each side, until golden. Heat berries in microwave for 30 to 45 seconds, mash with fork, and serve on French toast.

301 calories, 8 g total fat, 2 g saturated fat, 212 mg cholesterol, 458 mg sodium, 37 g carbohydrates, 7 g fiber, 20 g protein

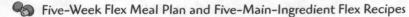

Zucchini-Spice-Pecan Pancakes

I have loved zucchini bread ever since childhood when my mom would make it with zucchini from our small backyard garden. This is a quicker pancake version, and it hits the spot when the craving hits.

- ⅓ cup *prepared* whole-grain pancake mix (such as Arrowhead Mills, Bob's Red Mill, or Krusteaz)
- ½ cup grated zucchini
- 2 tablespoons chopped pecans
- ½ teaspoon pie spice (apple or pumpkin)
- Cooking spray
- 1 teaspoon maple syrup

Mix batter, zucchini, pecans, and spice. Cook about three 4-inch pancakes on skillet sprayed with cooking spray. Drizzle lightly with syrup.

311 calories, 19 g total fat, 3 g saturated fat, 47 mg cholesterol, 396 mg sodium, 31 g carbohydrates, 5 g fiber, 8 g protein

Week Three Flex Lunches

Apple, Fennel, and Pistachio Salad

Fennel has a mild taste of licorice, but even if you don't like licorice (I don't), you will still love finely sliced fennel on this fresh and crunchy salad. The fennel makes the salad special—don't skip it.

1 apple, chopped
½ fennel bulb, thinly sliced
¼ cup chopped pistachios
3 cups green spring salad mix
2 tablespoons Universal Lemon-Flax Vinaigrette (see Index) or low-fat Italian dressing

Toss all ingredients together.

395 calories, 24 g total fat, 3 g saturated fat, 0 mg cholesterol, 163 mg sodium, 43 g carbohydrates, 13 g fiber, 11 g protein

Out and About

Never order anything directly off a restaurant menu. Always make healthy requests, such as hold the cheese and mayo, substitute baked chicken or fish for breaded or fried, swap a high-fat side dish like fries for the vegetable of the day, or ask for dressing on the side.

Greek Chopped Pita Salad

The pita is chopped into the salad for a fun and healthy take on croutons.

3 cups romaine lettuce, shredded
½ ounce feta cheese, crumbled
½ cup canned garbanzo beans, rinsed and drained
½ cucumber, chopped
2 tablespoons chopped fresh dill
1 whole-grain pita pocket, toasted and cut into bite-size pieces
2 tablespoons Universal Lemon-Flax Vinaigrette (see Index) or low-fat Italian dressing

Toss all ingredients together.

408 calories, 15 g total fat, 3 g saturated fat, 13 mg cholesterol, 404 mg sodium, 57 g carbohydrates, 13 g fiber, 16 g protein

Flex Swap ½ cup garbanzo beans with 2 ounces cooked, diced chicken breast.

Three-Bean Wrap with Maple Chili Sauce

Use any leftover canned beans you have for this recipe. I like using cannellini, kidney, and navy beans, but any combo is possible and will taste great in the sweet maple sauce with a subtle chili bite.

- 2 tablespoons ketchup
- 1 teaspoon maple syrup
- 1 teaspoon chili powder
- 1 clove garlic, minced
- ¾ cup canned beans, rinsed and drained (use a mixture of various beans)
- 1 small green bell pepper, finely chopped
- 2 small (6-inch) whole-grain tortillas

Mix first six ingredients together and heat in microwave for about 60 seconds. Wrap in tortillas. Heat in microwave for an additional 10 to 15 seconds.

387 calories, 2 g total fat, 0 g saturated fat, 0 mg cholesterol, 720 mg sodium, 88 g carbohydrates, 16 g fiber, 18 g protein

Southwest Guacamole Burger

Mashed avocado mixed with store-bought salsa makes a quick guacamole that is packed with heart-smart monounsaturated fat.

- ½ avocado, mashed
- 2 tablespoons salsa
- 2 tablespoons chopped fresh cilantro
- 1 vegetarian black-bean burger, heated
- 1 whole-grain hamburger bun

Mix mashed avocado with salsa and cilantro. Put hot burger on bun, and top with avocado mixture (guacamole).

409 calories, 21 g total fat, 3 g saturated fat, 0 mg cholesterol, 685 mg sodium, 42 g carbohydrates, 14 g fiber, 19 g protein

Out and About

Read between the lines. Certain words on a restaurant menu automatically warn you of a dish that is high in calories and fat, such as *fried, crispy, breaded, creamy, scalloped,* and *sautéed.* Look for healthy words instead, such as *broiled, baked, grilled, roasted, poached,* and *steamed.*

Beet and Goat Cheese Salad

I disliked beets until I ate a version of this salad in Wolfgang Puck's restaurant at the Contemporary Art Museum in Chicago. After making this beet salad a few times at home, I started loving beets! I prefer this with walnut oil, so use it if you have it.

2 tablespoons balsamic vinegar
2 teaspoons olive oil or walnut oil
3 cups green spring salad mix
¾ cup canned no-salt-added sliced beets, drained and quartered
1 ounce goat cheese, crumbled
3 tablespoons chopped walnuts

Toss together vinegar, oil, and greens. Top with beets, goat cheese, and walnuts.

396 calories, 30 g total fat, 7 g saturated fat, 13 mg cholesterol, 213 mg sodium, 22 g carbohydrates, 6 g fiber, 13 g protein

Out and About

Convenience versus socializing. Dine out only for *social occasions* (dates or nights out with your friends), and don't dine out just for *convenience*. If you want something convenient, warm up a frozen meal, heat a quick can of low-sodium soup with a whole-grain roll, or make a fast and healthy meal at home instead.

Roasted Red Pepper and Hummus Pita

Roasted red peppers in a jar (in water) are flavorful and have only 15 calories per ¼-cup serving.

- 1 whole-grain pita pocket, split in half
- ½ cup jarred (in water) roasted red peppers, drained
- 4 tablespoons hummus
- 1 cup low-sodium lentil soup (brands with less than 500 mg sodium per cup), heated

Stuff pita with red peppers and hummus. Serve with hot soup.

393 calories, 8 g total fat, 1 g saturated fat, 0 mg cholesterol, 794 mg sodium, 67 g carbohydrates, 14 g fiber, 17 g protein

Fact Stack

When you start a meal with soup, you automatically eat 100 total calories less per meal without even trying, because soup fills you up. Try minestrone before an Italian meal and miso soup before an Asian meal.

Pear and Swiss Sandwich

Sweet pear slices with a tart slice of Swiss and mustard make a "pear"-fect sandwich combo.

- 2 slices whole-grain bread, toasted
- 1 small pear, thinly sliced
- 1 slice (1 ounce) Swiss cheese
- 2 teaspoons mustard
- 1 cup green spring salad mix
- 1 tablespoon Universal Lemon-Flax Vinaigrette (see Index) or low-fat Italian dressing

Make a sandwich of toasted bread, pear, cheese, and mustard. Serve with salad tossed in vinaigrette.

395 calories, 15 g total fat, 6 g saturated fat, 26 mg cholesterol, 500 mg sodium, 54 g carbohydrates, 9 g fiber, 15 g protein

Flex Swap 1 slice Swiss cheese for 1 slice of vegetarian cheese.

Week Three Flex Dinners

Potatoes and Brussels Sprouts with Parmesan

This is a favorite recipe among my cooking-class participants—even those who didn't like brussels sprouts gleefully gobbled them down and went back for seconds.

1 cup brussels sprouts, cut in half
1 potato (with skin), cut into small 1- to 2-inch chunks
1 tablespoon olive oil
2 cloves garlic, minced
Dash of salt and black pepper
½ cup canned navy beans, rinsed and drained
2 tablespoons grated Parmesan cheese

Preheat oven to 400°F. Toss brussels sprouts, potatoes, oil, garlic, salt, and black pepper. Spread on cookie sheet and bake 30 to 40 minutes until vegetables are tender (occasionally shake pan to brown evenly). Add beans to cookie sheet for the last 15 minutes of baking. Top with Parmesan.

505 calories, 17 g total fat, 4 g saturated fat, 9 mg cholesterol, 342 mg sodium, 73 g carbohydrates, 16 g fiber, 19 g protein

Flex Swap ½ cup navy beans for 2 ounces of cooked, diced chicken breast.

Fried Beans and Garlic Greens

This dish was inspired by a trip I took to Greece. Going to Greece was one of my favorite culinary adventures because they use beans in so many of their recipes. Use the large, white Fordhook lima beans and not the smaller, green baby limas.

- 3 teaspoons olive oil, *split*
- ½ cup canned butter beans, rinsed and drained (Fordhook, large lima beans)
- 2 cloves garlic, minced
- Dash of crushed red pepper flakes
- 2 cups chopped Swiss chard
- 1 small whole-grain baguette or roll (about 4 inches), cut in half and toasted
- 1 tablespoon balsamic vinegar

Heat 1 teaspoon oil in skillet over medium heat, and panfry beans until slightly browned, about 8 minutes. Set aside. Sauté remaining 2 teaspoons oil, garlic, and red pepper for 1 minute. Add chard and cook until tender, 6 to 8 minutes. Serve cooked greens on toasted baguette, and top with fried beans and a drizzle of vinegar.

489 calories, 16 g total fat, 2 g saturated fat, 0 mg cholesterol, 627 mg sodium, 69 g carbohydrates, 9 g fiber, 17 g protein

Flex Swap ½ cup butter beans for 2 ounces cooked, diced low-fat chicken sausage.

Cauliflower-Cashew Curry

I didn't think I liked that bright yellow curry powder until I paired it with cauliflower, cashews, and raisins. Now when I meet people who also think they don't like curry, I ask them to try this. I have created many curry converts.

1 cup chopped cauliflower
1 teaspoon curry powder
½ cup crushed no-salt-added tomatoes (*not* drained)
½ cup canned kidney beans, rinsed and drained
¼ cup frozen peas, thawed
1 tablespoon raisins
¾ cup cooked brown rice (precooked microwavable or, if time allows, simmer your own)
2 tablespoons chopped cashews
1 green onion, chopped

In a medium saucepan over medium heat, cook cauliflower, curry powder, tomatoes, kidney beans, peas, and raisins covered for 10 to 12 minutes (stirring occasionally). Serve on brown rice, and top with cashews and green onion.

491 calories, 10 g total fat, 2 g saturated fat, 0 mg cholesterol, 98 mg sodium, 86 g carbohydrates, 19 g fiber, 20 g protein

Flex Swap ½ cup kidney beans for 2 ounces (9 medium) frozen cooked shrimp, thawed.

Black Beans and Fajita-Style Millet

This is a totally new twist on the classic bell pepper and onion fajitas.

½ cup water
¼ cup uncooked millet
1 clove garlic, minced
1 teaspoon cumin
1½ cups diced bell peppers of various colors (red, green, and yellow)
½ onion, diced
½ cup canned black beans, rinsed and drained
2 teaspoons olive oil
½ lime, juiced
2 tablespoons chopped cilantro
Dash of salt

Bring water and millet to a boil. Simmer (covered) for about 15 minutes, until water is absorbed. Sauté garlic, cumin, bell peppers, onion, and black beans in oil over medium heat. Combine pepper mixture with cooked millet, and top with lime juice, cilantro, and salt.

490 calories, 13 g total fat, 2 g saturated fat, 0 mg cholesterol, 178 mg sodium, 82 g carbohydrates, 15 g fiber, 17 g protein

Grilled Primavera Rigatoni

The colorful grilled vegetables add disease-fighting flavor to this recipe. Grill extra vegetables so you can put leftovers on sandwiches and in pitas.

- ¾ cup (2 ounces) uncooked whole-grain rigatoni
- ½ small zucchini, sliced thick
- ½ small red onion, sliced thick
- ½ small yellow squash, sliced thick
- 2 plum tomatoes, halved
- 2 teaspoons olive oil
- 1 teaspoon dried rosemary
- Dash of salt and black pepper
- ¼ cup canned cannellini beans, rinsed and drained
- 1 tablespoon pine nuts

Cook pasta al dente according to package directions. Toss together zucchini, onion, squash, tomatoes, oil, rosemary, salt, and black pepper. Grill ingredients indoors on grill pan or on outdoor grill for 10 minutes (turning once), until tender with light grill marks. Toss together cooked pasta, grilled vegetables, and beans. Top with pine nuts.

514 calories, 17 g total fat, 2 g saturated fat, 0 mg cholesterol, 198 mg sodium, 81 g carbohydrates, 15 g fiber, 18 g protein

Spicy Tofu Reuben

I have to give credit to my husband for this one. This was one of his first attempts at making something with veggie white meat, and it really tastes great!

1 slice (3 ounces) extra-firm tofu (press to remove excess water)
1 teaspoon olive oil
2 tablespoons light canola mayonnaise (such as eggless Spectrum)
1 tablespoon ketchup
1 tablespoon sweet relish
Dash or two of hot sauce
2 slices whole-grain bread, toasted
3 tablespoons canned or refrigerated sauerkraut
1 slice Swiss cheese

Sauté tofu slice in oil over medium heat for 5 to 6 minutes on each side, until golden. Mix mayonnaise, ketchup, relish, and hot sauce, and spread on toasted bread. Make sandwich with golden tofu, sauerkraut, and Swiss cheese.

499 calories, 27 g total fat, 8 g saturated fat, 33 mg cholesterol, 865 mg sodium, 45 g carbohydrates, 5 g fiber, 25 g protein

Flex Swap 3 ounces tofu for 3 ounces sliced turkey breast.

Italian Spaghetti Squash

After spaghetti squash is baked, the flesh becomes a delicious stand-in for angel hair pasta with only 42 calories per cup (four times fewer calories than pasta). My dad is a big fan of this one.

½ spaghetti squash
1 teaspoon olive oil
1 clove garlic, minced
½ cup canned navy beans, rinsed and drained
1 leek (white part only), thinly sliced
½ cup canned no-salt-added crushed tomatoes (not drained)
1 tablespoon Italian seasoning
1 tablespoon balsamic vinegar
2 tablespoons grated Parmesan cheese

Remove seeds from ½ spaghetti squash. Put flesh side down on a plate, and microwave for 12 to 15 minutes or cook in 350°F oven on cookie sheet for 30 minutes. Sauté oil, garlic, beans, leek, tomatoes, seasoning, and vinegar for 7 to 10 minutes over medium heat. When squash is tender, use fork to pull out the spaghetti-like strands, and discard hollowed-out shell. Top spaghetti-like squash strands with bean mixture. Sprinkle with Parmesan cheese.

481 calories, 10 g total fat, 3 g saturated fat, 9 mg cholesterol, 209 mg sodium, 84 g carbohydrates, 22 g fiber, 18 g protein

Flex Swap ½ cup navy beans with 2 ounces cooked chicken breast.

Week Three Flex Snacks and Desserts

Tomato Juice Cocktail and Chickpea Nuts

When you bake chickpeas in a hot oven, a miracle happens—they become the best-tasting cocktail nut around!

½ cup canned garbanzo beans, rinsed, drained, and pat dry
¼ teaspoon chili powder
Dash of salt and black pepper
6 ounces low-sodium tomato juice

Preheat oven to 375°F. Toss garbanzo beans with chili powder, salt, and black pepper. Place garbanzo beans on cookie sheet, and bake for about 30 minutes (shake occasionally to brown evenly). They will be firm and crunchy like a nut. Serve with tomato juice.

149 calories, 2 g total fat, 0 g saturated fat, 0 mg cholesterol, 287 mg sodium, 27 g carbohydrates, 7 g fiber, 7 g protein

Note: Make extra chickpea nuts to have on hand for the week.

Peanut Butter and Celery

A simple snack is sometimes all you want and all you have time for.

1½ tablespoons peanut butter
4 celery stalks

152 calories, 12 g total fat, 2 g saturated fat, 0 mg cholesterol, 165 mg sodium, 7 g carbohydrates, 3 g fiber, 6 g protein

Fact Stack

Fill up with wet foods. Foods with a high percentage of water such as fruits, vegetables, soup, and oatmeal make you feel fuller than do dry foods such as toast, crackers, or chips.

Swiss and Crispbread

Crackers and cheese are a classic and satisfying snack combo. Be mindful to keep portions to 150 calories by portioning the crackers and cheese on a plate rather than eating them straight from the package.

1 slice (1 ounce) Swiss cheese
2 whole-grain crispbread crackers (e.g., Wasa)

154 calories, 9 g total fat, 5 g saturated fat, 26 mg cholesterol, 130 mg sodium, 10 g carbohydrates, 1 g fiber, 9 g protein

Flex Swap 1 slice Swiss cheese with 1 slice vegetarian cheese.

Fact Stack

Table, plate, chair—always use these three things when you eat meals and snacks. Research shows that you'll eat 43 percent smaller portions if you eat at a *table,* sitting in a *chair* and eating from a *plate* rather than eating out of the fridge standing in the kitchen or on the couch in the living room in front of the television.

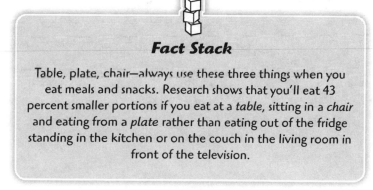

Grape, Almond, and Mint Salad

It may seem an unlikely combination, but the three flavors complement each other deliciously. This is a perfect subtly sweet after-meal treat because mint helps digestion.

1 cup halved red grapes
2 tablespoons chopped fresh mint
2 tablespoons sliced almonds
1 tablespoon white balsamic vinegar
Dash of salt

Toss all ingredients together.

142 calories, 7 g total fat, 1 g saturated fat, 0 mg cholesterol, 158 mg sodium, 20 g carbohydrates, 3 g fiber, 3 g protein

Craving Control

Make your dentist proud. Brush your teeth after meals to decrease the automatic postmeal need for something sweet. Also try mint gum or mint tea as research suggests the smell of mint can help reduce your weekly calories by as much as 23 percent.

Almond-Stuffed Dates

Dates are super sticky and sweet—they are a natural way to treat a sweet tooth.

- 5 dates, pitted
- 5 whole almonds

Stuff almonds into dates.

152 calories, 3 g total fat, 0 g saturated fat, 0 mg cholesterol, 1 mg sodium, 32 g carbohydrates, 4 g fiber, 2 g protein

Out and About

Arm's length away. Socialize away from the food table at parties and gatherings. The farther away you stand, the less you will nibble.

Dark-Chocolate-Dipped Apricots

These are as pretty as they are delicious. Any time I bring them to parties, they are one of the first things to go. Package them in a pretty tin, and they are a perfect hostess gift.

2 tablespoons dark chocolate chips
2 dried apricots
2 teaspoons crushed pistachios

Melt chocolate chips (using a microwave or double boiler). Dip apricots in chocolate, covering only 50 percent of apricot. Sprinkle with crushed pistachios. Place on wax paper to set, about 10 minutes.

154 calories, 9 g total fat, 4 g saturated fat, 0 mg cholesterol, 3 mg sodium, 20 g carbohydrates, 2 g fiber, 2 g protein

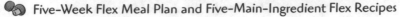

Sweet Cocoa Yogurt

Unsweetened cocoa has only 7 calories per teaspoon and is rich in disease-fighting cocoa flavonoids. You will enjoy this deep, rich chocolate-mousse-like treat.

1 container (6 ounce) low-fat plain yogurt
1 teaspoon unsweetened cocoa powder
2 teaspoons agave nectar

Mix yogurt, cocoa powder, and agave together.

151 calories, 3 g total fat, 2 g saturated fat, 10 mg cholesterol, 119 mg sodium, 24 g carbohydrates, 1 g fiber, 9 g protein

Week Three Flex Shopping List

Make sure you have your fridge, pantry, and spice rack staples stocked (pages 79–80). Amounts in parentheses indicate how much you will use this week.

This list is for one person; multiply the ingredients if you are cooking for more. Check off what you need from the grocery store this week.

Grains

- ☐ Baguette or bread roll, whole grain (1 small)
- ☐ Bread, whole grain (6 slices)
- ☐ Brown rice (¾ cups precooked microwavable or ¼ cup uncooked)
- ☐ Bulgur (¼ cup uncooked)
- ☐ Cereal, cold, whole grain (1 cup)
- ☐ Crispbread crackers, whole grain (2 crackers such as Wasa)
- ☐ Hamburger bun, whole grain (1)
- ☐ Millet (¼ cup uncooked)
- ☐ Oats, rolled (1 cup)
- ☐ Pancake mix, whole grain (⅓ cup prepared)
- ☐ Pita pocket, whole grain (2)
- ☐ Rigatoni, whole grain (¾ cup uncooked = 2 ounces uncooked)
- ☐ Tortillas, whole grain (2 small)

Fruit

- ☐ 100 percent apple juice (¼ cup)
- ☐ Apples (2)
- ☐ Apricots, dried (2)
- ☐ Avocado (1)
- ☐ Banana (1)
- ☐ Blueberries (1 cup)
- ☐ Cranberries, dried (2 tablespoons)
- ☐ Dates (5)
- ☐ Pear (1)
- ☐ Raisins (3 tablespoons)
- ☐ Red grapes (1 cup)
- ☐ Strawberries (¾ cup)

Fresh Herbs and Flavorings

- ☐ Cilantro, fresh (4 tablespoons)
- ☐ Dill, fresh (4 tablespoons)
- ☐ Mint, fresh (2 tablespoons)

Vegetables

- ☐ Bell pepper, green (1 pepper + ½ cup diced)
- ☐ Bell pepper, red (½ cup diced)
- ☐ Bell pepper, yellow (½ cup diced)
- ☐ Broccoli (1 cup)
- ☐ Brussels sprouts (1 cup)
- ☐ Cauliflower (1 cup)
- ☐ Celery (4 stalks)
- ☐ Cucumber (½)
- ☐ Fennel bulb (½)
- ☐ Green onions (1)
- ☐ Green spring salad mix (7 cups)
- ☐ Leek (1)
- ☐ Plum tomatoes (2)
- ☐ Potato (1)
- ☐ Romaine lettuce (3 cups)
- ☐ Spaghetti squash (½)
- ☐ Swiss chard (2 cups)
- ☐ Yellow squash (½)
- ☐ Zucchini (1)

Nuts, Seeds, and Miscellaneous

- ☐ Agave nectar (2 teaspoons)
- ☐ Almonds (5 whole and 2 tablespoons sliced)
- ☐ Cashews (2 tablespoons chopped)
- ☐ Cocoa powder, unsweetened (1 teaspoon)
- ☐ Dark chocolate chips, semisweet (2 tablespoons)
- ☐ Hot sauce (1 to 2 dashes)
- ☐ Mayonnaise, light canola (2 tablespoons)
- ☐ Pecans (2 tablespoons chopped)
- ☐ Pine nuts (1 tablespoon)

- ☐ Pistachios (about 5 tablespoons shelled)
- ☐ Sweet relish (1 tablespoon)
- ☐ Walnuts (4 tablespoons chopped)

Refrigerated Products

- ☐ Eggs (2 whole + 5 whites)
- ☐ Feta cheese (½ ounce)
- ☐ Goat cheese (1 ounce)
- ☐ Hummus (4 tablespoons)
- ☐ Parmesan cheese (4 tablespoons, grated)
- ☐ Plain yogurt, low fat (½ cup + 6-ounce container)
- ☐ Swiss cheese (4 slices)
- ☐ Tofu, extra firm (3 ounces)

Canned and Frozen Goods

- ☐ Beets, canned no-salt-added and sliced (¾ cup)
- ☐ Black beans, canned (½ cup)
- ☐ Butter beans or large Fordhook lima beans, canned (½ cup)
- ☐ Cannellini beans, canned (½ cup)
- ☐ Garbanzo beans, canned (1 cup)
- ☐ Kidney beans, canned (¾ cup)
- ☐ Lentil soup, low sodium (1 cup)
- ☐ Navy beans, canned (1¼ cups)
- ☐ Roasted red bell peppers, jarred in water (½ cup)
- ☐ Sauerkraut, canned or refrigerated (3 tablespoons)
- ☐ Tomato juice, low sodium (6 ounces)
- ☐ Frozen mixed berries, unsweetened (⅓ cup)
- ☐ Frozen peas (¼ cup)
- ☐ Veggie burger, black bean (1)

Week Four Recipes, Meal Plan, Shopping List

Week Four Flex Breakfasts

Pumpkin-Spice Oatmeal with Hazelnuts

Pumpkin is one of my favorite oatmeal toppings. Hazelnuts taste great with pumpkin and are one of the seven nuts the U.S. Food and Drug Administration classifies as heart healthy (the other six are almonds, peanuts, pecans, pine nuts, pistachios, and walnuts).

- ½ cup skim milk or soy milk
- ½ cup water
- ½ cup rolled oats
- ¼ cup canned pumpkin
- ½ teaspoon pie spice (apple or pumpkin)
- 1 tablespoon chopped hazelnuts
- 2 teaspoons agave nectar

Bring milk, water, and oats to a boil. Simmer and stir for 5 minutes. Stir in pumpkin and spice. Top with nuts and agave nectar.

301 calories, 7 g total fat, 1 g saturated fat, 2 mg cholesterol, 61 mg sodium, 49 g carbohydrates, 7 g fiber, 12 g protein

Honey, Pear, and Almond Muesli

I fell in love with muesli (uncooked oats with fruit and nuts) when I was visiting Germany for a nutrition conference. Typically it is lower in calories and sugar than granola. I like to soak my oats for 10 minutes or overnight to make it a tender, almost-cooked consistency.

- ½ cup rolled oats
- ½ cup skim milk or soy milk
- ½ small pear, chopped
- 1 tablespoon sliced almonds, toasted
- 1 teaspoon honey

Mix *raw* oats with milk. Stir in pear, almonds, and honey. Let sit 10 minutes or overnight in fridge.

299 calories, 6 g total fat, 1 g saturated fat, 2 mg cholesterol, 54 mg sodium, 52 g carbohydrates, 7 g fiber, 12 g protein

Typical Breakfast with Refried Black Beans

This recipe was inspired by the breakfasts I ate on my honeymoon in Honduras.

1 whole egg + 2 egg whites
Cooking spray
⅓ cup canned low-fat refried black beans
1 small (6-inch) whole-grain tortilla
2 tablespoons shredded part-skim mozzarella cheese
Dash of hot sauce

Scramble egg and egg whites in pan sprayed with cooking spray. Heat beans separately in microwave for about 30 to 45 seconds. Spread beans into tortilla, and fill with eggs, cheese, and hot sauce.

287 calories, 9 g total fat, 3 g saturated fat, 219 mg cholesterol, 548 mg sodium, 33 g carbohydrates, 5 g fiber, 24 g protein

Flex Swap 1 whole egg + 2 eggs whites with ½ cup chopped firm tofu sautéed with ⅛ teaspoon turmeric (for yellow color).

Peaches and Candied-Ginger Yogurt

I include this recipe as a breakfast option, but it easily can be transformed into a dessert. For dessert, grill or broil a fresh peach half, drizzle on 1 tablespoon of plain yogurt, and sprinkle with 1 tablespoon of chopped candied ginger.

¼ cup rolled oats
2 teaspoons honey
1 container (6 ounce) plain low-fat yogurt
1 peach, diced
2 tablespoons chopped candied ginger

Toast oats in dry pan until golden. Stir honey into yogurt, and top with peaches, toasted oats, and ginger.

299 calories, 2 g total fat, 0 g saturated fat, 3 mg cholesterol, 132 mg sodium, 59 g carbohydrates, 4 g fiber, 15 g protein

Green Apple and Sunflower Seed Butter Toast

I can't say much more than "Yum." I love this with sunflower seed butter (also known as SunButter), but if you don't have it, you can use peanut or almond butter instead.

- 1½ tablespoons sunflower seed butter
- 1 slice whole-grain bread, toasted
- 1 green apple, thinly sliced

Spread sunflower seed butter on toast. Top with green apple slices.

291 calories, 14 g total fat, 2 g saturated fat, 0 mg cholesterol, 140 mg sodium, 39 g carbohydrates, 5 g fiber, 8 g protein

Waffles with Maple-Berry Compote

Most waffle and pancake syrups are merely processed high-fructose corn syrup. Pour on nutrition by making your own syrup made mostly of mashed berries and just a hint of natural 100 percent maple syrup.

½ cup unsweetened frozen mixed berries, thawed
1 tablespoon maple syrup
2 frozen whole-grain waffles, toasted

Mash berries with syrup, heat in microwave for 30 seconds, and put on top of toasted waffles.

300 calories, 9 g total fat, 2 g saturated fat, 70 mg cholesterol, 368 mg sodium, 50 g carbohydrates, 6 g fiber, 8 g protein

Breakfast Fajitas

Red, green, and yellow bell peppers sautéed with garlic, onions, and a squeeze of lime perk up tired scrambled eggs.

½ cup sliced bell peppers of various colors (red, green, and yellow)
¼ cup sliced onion
1 teaspoon olive oil
½ teaspoon cumin
Dash of salt and black pepper
1 whole egg + 2 egg whites
1 small (6-inch) whole-grain tortilla
½ grapefruit

Sauté peppers, onion, olive oil, cumin, salt, and black pepper for 3 to 5 minutes and set aside. Scramble eggs, and wrap them in tortilla with bell peppers and onion. Serve grapefruit on the side.

298 calories, 11 g total fat, 2 g saturated fat, 212 mg cholesterol, 510 mg sodium, 40 g carbohydrates, 5 g fiber, 18 g protein

Flex Swap 1 whole egg + 2 egg whites with ½ cup crumbled firm tofu sauteéd with ⅛ teaspoon turmeric (for yellow color).

Week Four Flex Lunches

Spicy Peanut and Edamame Wrap

I am a sucker for anything with peanut sauce, and this version could not be easier. You can also use the sauce in other ways such as on fresh broccoli or cauliflower.

1 tablespoon peanut butter
1 teaspoon sesame oil
2 tablespoons rice vinegar
Dash of crushed red pepper flakes
½ cup shelled frozen edamame, thawed
½ cup shredded carrots
2 small (6-inch) whole-grain tortillas

Whisk together peanut butter, oil, vinegar, and red pepper. Toss with edamame and carrots, and wrap mixture in tortillas. Heat in microwave for 30 to 45 seconds.

402 calories, 18 g total fat, 3 g saturated fat, 0 mg cholesterol, 459 mg sodium, 58 g carbohydrates, 10 g fiber, 19 g protein

Pinto Bean Lunch Tacos

Lunchtime tacos will get you out of the same-old-sandwich funk.

- 3/4 cup canned pinto beans, drained and rinsed
- 1/4 cup salsa
- 2 tablespoons low-fat sour cream
- 1 cup romaine lettuce, shredded
- 2 small (6-inch) whole-grain tortillas

Toss pinto beans, salsa, and sour cream together. Put bean mixture and lettuce in tortillas, and wrap.

395 calories, 5 g total fat, 2 g saturated fat, 11 mg cholesterol, 538 mg sodium, 81 g carbohydrates, 18 g fiber, 20 g protein

Flex Swap 2 tablespoons low-fat sour cream with 2 tablespoons sour cream.

Bay Avocado Sandwich

This recipe was inspired by a lunch I had on my honeymoon in Honduras. It will be the freshest-tasting meal you've ever had.

- 1 teaspoon Old Bay seasoning
- 1 lime, juiced
- 1 teaspoon olive oil
- ¼ avocado, diced
- ½ cup canned garbanzo beans, rinsed, drained, and chopped
- ¼ cup finely chopped red bell pepper
- 1 celery stalk, finely chopped
- 1 green onion, finely chopped
- 1 small whole-grain roll, removing center of bread to leave more room for filling

Whisk Old Bay with lime juice and oil. Toss together with remaining ingredients, and spoon into roll.

415 calories, 17 g total fat, 2 g saturated fat, 0 mg cholesterol, 230 mg sodium, 59 g carbohydrates, 15 g fiber, 14 g protein

Flex Swap ½ cup garbanzo beans with 2 ounces cooked, diced chicken breast.

Monster Black-Bean Burger

Coleslaw piled high makes this burger a monster. It is inspired by my husband's favorite meal at a vegetarian-friendly restaurant in Chicago called Earwax Café.

1 cup broccoli coleslaw (Mann's brand)
1 tablespoon Universal Lemon-Flax Vinaigrette (see Index) or low-fat Italian dressing
1 black-bean burger, heated
1 tablespoon barbecue sauce
1 whole-grain hamburger bun
1 plum

Toss broccoli coleslaw with vinaigrette. Top hot burger with dressed coleslaw and barbecue sauce. Serve on bun with plum on the side.

390 calories, 12 g total fat, 1 g saturated fat, 2 mg cholesterol, 739 mg sodium, 56 g carbohydrates, 12 g fiber, 19 g protein

Egg Salad Sandwich

I use light canola mayo in this lunchtime classic. Try substituting tofu in place of the eggs for an eggless egg salad!

1 whole hard-boiled egg + 2 hard-boiled egg whites, chopped
1 tablespoon light canola mayonnaise (such as eggless Spectrum)
2 teaspoons prepared mustard
1 stalk celery, chopped fine
1/4 cup finely chopped cucumber
Dash of black pepper
2 slices whole-grain bread
1 apple

Mix first six ingredients together, and serve on bread with apple on the side.

382 calories, 11 g total fat, 3 g saturated fat, 215 mg cholesterol, 693 mg sodium, 54 g carbohydrates, 8 g fiber, 21 g protein

Flex Swap 1 whole eggs + 2 egg whites for 1/2 cup crumbled firm tofu mixed with 1/8 teaspoon turmeric (for yellow color).

Artichoke and White-Bean Hummus Pita

Often I will just buy the hummus already made from the store, but this version is worth taking the time to make the hummus yourself.

- 1/4 cup chopped onion
- 1 teaspoon Italian seasoning
- 1/8 teaspoon crushed red pepper flakes
- 1 teaspoon olive oil
- 1/2 cup canned Great Northern beans, drained and rinsed
- 1/2 cup canned (in water) artichoke hearts, drained
- 1/2 lemon, juiced
- 1/2 cup cucumber, sliced
- 1 whole-grain pita pocket, cut in half

Sauté onion, Italian seasoning, and red pepper flakes in olive oil for about 5 minutes. In a large bowl, using a hand blender, puree cooked onion, beans, artichoke hearts, and lemon juice until smooth. Stuff mixture and cucumbers into pita halves.

387 calories, 8 g total fat, 1 g saturated fat, 0 mg cholesterol, 461 mg sodium, 69 g carbohydrates, 20 g fiber, 17 g protein

"Chicken" Ranch Salad

This is definitely a fast and favorite meal of mine. When I have 5 minutes or less, this recipe is a perfect solution.

- 1 teaspoon ranch seasoning
- 2 tablespoons Universal Lemon-Flax Vinaigrette (see Index) or low-fat Italian dressing
- 1 vegetarian "chicken" patty, chopped
- ½ cup cherry tomatoes, halved
- ¼ cup canned no-salt-added corn, drained
- ¼ cup chopped green bell pepper
- 3 cups green spring salad mix
- 1 nectarine

Whisk ranch seasoning into vinaigrette. Toss all salad ingredients together. Serve with nectarine on the side.

396 calories, 16 g total fat, 2 g saturated fat, 2 mg cholesterol, 573 mg sodium, 52 g carbohydrates, 12 g fiber, 19 g protein

Flex Swap vegetarian chicken patty for 3 ounces cooked, diced chicken.

Week Four Flex Dinners

Pinto and Cheese Poblanos

Poblano peppers have a little heat but are fairly mild. Just be sure to take out the veins and seeds to decrease the spice. Quinoa works well in all types of stuffed-pepper dishes.

½ cup water
¼ cup uncooked quinoa
¾ cup canned pinto beans, rinsed and drained
2 tablespoons shredded cheddar cheese
1 teaspoon cumin
2 poblano peppers, left whole with veins and seeds removed

Bring water and quinoa to a boil. Simmer (covered) for 15 minutes. Stir beans, cheese, and cumin into cooked quinoa. Stuff peppers with filling, and broil on cookie sheet for 15 minutes, turning periodically until browned on all sides.

490 calories, 13 g total fat, 6 g saturated fat, 30 mg cholesterol, 197 mg sodium, 70 g carbohydrates, 16 g fiber, 26 g protein

Flex Swap ¾ cup pinto beans for 3 ounces cooked extra-lean ground turkey or sirloin.

Cilantro-Peanut Stir-Fry

Frozen vegetables save time because they are already cut and cleaned. The peanut flavor comes from peanut oil and tastes great with fresh cilantro.

- ½ cup extra-firm tofu (pressed to remove excess water)
- 2 teaspoons peanut oil, *split*
- 2 cups frozen stir-fry mixed vegetables
- ½-inch chunk ginger, grated
- 2 cloves garlic, minced
- ¼ cup 100 percent pineapple juice
- 1 cup cooked brown rice (precooked microwavable or, if time allows, simmer your own)
- 2 tablespoons chopped cilantro

Cut tofu into ½-inch cubes. Sauté tofu in 1 teaspoon oil over medium heat about 10 minutes (stirring only two to three times) until golden, and set aside. Sauté vegetables in remaining 1 teaspoon oil, ginger, garlic, and pineapple juice about 8 minutes, until tender. Heat microwavable brown rice. Serve stir-fried tofu and veggies on brown rice. Top with cilantro.

491 calories, 17 g total fat, 2 g saturated fat, 0 mg cholesterol, 64 mg sodium, 72 g carbohydrates, 10 g fiber, 19 g protein

Flex Swap ½ cup tofu for 2 ounces cooked chicken breast or lean steak strips.

Tuscan Bean Soup

My favorite soup, this recipe is a hands-down must-try. Drizzling the vinegar on top is a step that can't be skipped.

- ½ sweet yellow onion, diced
- 1 clove garlic, minced
- ½ teaspoon dried rosemary, crushed
- 1 teaspoon olive oil
- 1 cup canned garbanzo beans, rinsed and drained
- ½ cup canned no-salt-added diced tomatoes, (*not* drained)
- 1 cup water
- 2 tablespoons balsamic vinegar (topping)
- 1 small whole-grain roll

In medium pot, sauté onion, garlic, and rosemary in oil over medium heat for 3 minutes. Add beans, tomatoes, and water, bring to a boil, and simmer for 10 minutes. Put hand blender into pot, and blend soup to a semichunky texture. Serve with drizzled vinegar on top and whole-grain roll on the side for dipping.

489 calories, 10 g total fat, 1 g saturated fat, 0 mg cholesterol, 214 mg sodium, 84 g carbohydrates, 17 g fiber, 20 g protein

Sage-Butternut-Squash Pilaf

You aren't supposed to play favorites, but butternut squash has got to be one of mine. Pairing it with sage gives it a hint of stuffinglike flavor. You can buy precut butternut squash to save time.

- 1½ cups cut butternut squash (1-inch cubes)
- 2 teaspoons olive oil, *split*
- Dash of salt and black pepper
- ½ cup canned navy beans, rinsed and drained
- 1 teaspoon dried sage
- ½ cup cooked brown rice (precooked microwavable or, if time allows, simmer your own)
- 1 tablespoon chopped pecans

Preheat oven to 400°F. Toss squash with 1 teaspoon olive oil, salt, and black pepper. Bake on cookie sheet for 20 minutes (turning once). Sauté beans, sage, and cooked rice in remaining 1 teaspoon olive oil over medium heat. Combine baked butternut squash, bean-and-rice mixture, and pecans.

486 calories, 16 g total fat, 2 g saturated fat, 0 mg cholesterol, 165 mg sodium, 77 g carbohydrates, 17 g fiber, 13 g protein

Flex Swap ½ cup navy beans for 2 ounces cooked chicken breast.

BBQ Sandwich and Parsnip Fries

This healthy version of a McDonald's McRib Sandwich and the parsnip fries will easily become a family-favorite side dish.

- 2 medium parsnips, peeled and cut into french-fry shapes
- 1 teaspoon olive oil
- Dash of salt and black pepper
- ½ onion, sliced
- 2 tablespoons barbecue sauce
- 1 slice (2 ounces) tempeh (¼ of 8-ounce package)
- 1 whole-grain hamburger bun
- 3 dill pickle slices

Preheat oven to 400°F. Toss parsnips in oil, salt, and black pepper. Bake on cookie sheet for about 25 minutes, flipping once. Sauté onion slices, barbecue sauce, and tempeh over medium heat for 8 minutes. Serve tempeh and onions on bun topped with pickles. Serve with parsnip fries.

493 calories, 14 g total fat, 2 g saturated fat, 0 mg cholesterol, 62 mg sodium, 80 g carbohydrates, 16 g fiber, 19 g protein

Flex Swap 2 ounces of tempeh for 2 ounces sliced turkey breast.

Yellow Rice and Grilled Bok Choy

A dash of curry powder turns brown rice a magical yellow color—magical because the compounds in curry powder have disease-fighting powers such as protection against certain types of cancer (especially colon and skin), heart disease, and arthritis.

1 baby bok choy, cut in half
2 teaspoons olive oil, *split*
1 clove garlic, minced
¼ teaspoon curry powder
⅛ teaspoon cumin
Pinch of cinnamon
1 cup cooked brown rice (precooked microwavable or, if time allows, simmer your own)
½ cup canned black beans, rinsed and drained

Toss bok choy with 1 teaspoon oil and garlic. Grill (on indoor grill pan or outdoor grill) 5 minutes, flipping once. Sauté curry, cumin, cinnamon, cooked brown rice, and black beans in remaining 1 teaspoon olive oil over medium heat. Serve grilled bok choy on rice and beans.

491 calories, 12 g total fat, 2 g saturated fat, 0 mg cholesterol, 334 mg sodium, 81 g carbohydrates, 14 g fiber, 20 g protein

Flex Swap ½ cup black beans for 2 ounces cooked salmon, tuna, or other fish.

Caribbean Black Bean Couscous

I like mangos, and this is a savory way to enjoy their unique flavor. This is one of the most colorful meals you will ever eat.

¼ cup uncooked whole wheat couscous
½ cup water
¾ cup canned black beans, rinsed and drained
½ mango, diced
½ red bell pepper, diced
3 green onions, diced
1 jalapeño pepper, minced without veins or seeds
1 lime, juiced
1 teaspoon olive oil

Bring couscous and water to a boil. Take off from heat, cover for 15 minutes, and then fluff with fork. Warm beans in microwave for 1 to 2 minutes. Toss all ingredients with warm couscous.

495 calories, 6 g total fat, 1 g saturated fat, 0 mg cholesterol, 20 mg sodium, 96 g carbohydrates, 14 g fiber, 19 g protein

Week Four Flex Snacks and Desserts

Guacamole and Chips

I replace one avocado with a half-can of cannellini beans to save more than 100 calories per recipe.

- ¼ cup Guacamole (see following recipe)
- 7 whole-grain tortilla chips

Make guacamole. Serve dip with chips.

156 calories, 8 g total fat, 1 g saturated fat, 0 mg cholesterol, 104 mg sodium, 19 g carbohydrates, 6 g fiber, 4 g protein

Guacamole

Makes about 6 servings (¼ cup each)

- ¾ cup cannellini beans, rinsed and drained
- 1 avocado
- 1 plum tomato, chopped
- ½ lime, juiced
- ½ small onion, chopped
- 1 clove garlic, minced
- ¼ teaspoon of salt

Using hand blender, puree beans until smooth. Add avocado and mash together with fork until smooth. Stir in tomato, lime juice, onion, garlic, and salt. Keep tightly covered with plastic wrap in fridge for about three days.

Carrot Chips and Almond Butter

This is one of my favorite food combinations. I could eat it every day.

¾ cup cut carrots ("chip" shapes) or baby carrots
1 tablespoon almond butter

Spread almond butter on carrots.

139 calories, 10 g total fat, 1 g saturated fat, 0 mg cholesterol, 65 mg sodium, 12 g carbohydrates, 3 g fiber, 3 g protein

Out and About

Limit the variety of your selections when eating buffet-style. If you're at a party or gathering where food is served buffet-style, limit the number of items you put on your plate. Research shows that having many flavors at one meal can stimulate our appetite, but decreasing variety helps us feel full and satisfied with less food.

Honey-Whipped Cottage Cheese with Berries

If you don't have time to blend the cottage cheese you can eat it as is, but whipping it smooth makes it special. For a thicker texture, drain the cottage cheese before blending.

½ cup low-fat cottage cheese
2 teaspoons honey
¼ cup frozen unsweetened mixed berries, thawed

With hand blender, whip cottage cheese and honey until smooth. Serve with berries.

145 calories, 1 g total fat, 1 g saturated fat, 5 mg cholesterol, 16 mg sodium, 20 g carbohydrates, 1 g fiber, 14 g protein

Light Beer and Peanuts

You don't have to be watching a baseball game to enjoy this classic snack combo. If you don't drink alcohol, double your serving of peanuts and opt for a fruit juice spritzer instead.

1 light beer (12 ounces)
10 peanuts, in shell

156 calories, 5 g total fat, 1 g saturated fat, 0 mg cholesterol, 54 mg sodium, 8 g carbohydrates, 1 g fiber, 3 g protein

Craving Control

Try a fruit juice spritzer. Combine *8 ounces of club soda* with a *1½-ounce shot of 100 percent juice.* This naturally flavored beverage sips in at 25 to 30 calories. Use any flavor of 100 percent juice such as pomegranate, cherry, or grape.

Peach-Raspberry Crepe

The combo of peaches and raspberries has long been appreciated and is often called a peach melba. To save time, buy ready-made crepes (about 30 to 50 calories each) in the produce section of the store. Or you can make your own using 2 tablespoons whole-grain pancake batter + 2 tablespoons soy milk.

2 teaspoons raspberry 100 percent fruit spread or jam
¼ cup low-fat cottage cheese
1 ready-made crepe (such as Melissa's brand)
½ cup diced peaches (fresh or canned with no sugar added)

Mix jam and cottage cheese together and spread on crepe. Fill with peaches and roll.

151 calories, 3 g total fat, 1 g saturated fat, 37 mg cholesterol, 297 mg sodium, 21 g carbohydrates, 2 g fiber, 10 g protein

Pineapple with Candied Ginger and Pecans

This was voted one of the best desserts in my cooking class. I grill the pineapple to bring out even more natural sugars and sweet flavor. Bromelain, a natural enzyme in pineapple, and ginger both help with postmeal digestion.

- 3 pineapple rings (fresh or canned in own juice)
- 2 teaspoons chopped pecans
- 2 teaspoons chopped candied ginger

Top pineapple rings with pecans and ginger. For even more sweetness, grill pineapple rings before topping with pecans and ginger.

145 calories, 4 g total fat, 0 g saturated fat, 0 mg cholesterol, 2 mg sodium, 30 g carbohydrates, 2 g fiber, 1 g protein

Honey-Drizzled Yogurt

I prefer to get plain, unsweetened yogurt and add sweetness with either chopped fresh fruit or a little honey. One teaspoon of honey adds 21 calories and about 6 grams of sugar, which is still fewer calories and less sugar than the presweetened versions.

1 container (6 ounces) plain low-fat yogurt
2 teaspoons honey

Drizzle and stir honey into yogurt.

138 calories, 0 g total fat, 0 g saturated fat, 3 mg cholesterol, 131 mg sodium, 25 g carbohydrates, 0 g fiber, 10 g protein

Week Four Flex Shopping List

Make sure you have your fridge, pantry, and spice rack staples stocked (pages 79–80). Amounts in parentheses indicate how much you will use this week.

This list is for one person; multiply the ingredients if you are cooking for more. Check off what you need from the grocery store this week.

Grains

- ☐ Bread, whole grain (3 slices)
- ☐ Bread rolls, whole grain (2)
- ☐ Brown rice (2½ cups precooked microwavable or about 1 cup uncooked)
- ☐ Couscous, whole wheat (¼ cup uncooked)
- ☐ Hamburger buns, whole grain (2)
- ☐ Oats, rolled (1¼ cups)
- ☐ Pita pocket, whole grain (1)
- ☐ Quinoa (¼ cup uncooked)
- ☐ Tortillas, whole grain (6 small)

Fruit

- ☐ 100 percent pineapple juice (¼ cup)
- ☐ Apples (2)
- ☐ Avocados (2)
- ☐ Grapefruit (1)
- ☐ Mango (1)
- ☐ Nectarine (1)
- ☐ Peaches (2)
- ☐ Pears (1)
- ☐ Plum (1)

Fresh Herbs and Flavorings

- ☐ Cilantro, fresh (2 tablespoons)
- ☐ Ginger (½-inch chunk)

Vegetables

- ☐ Baby bok choy (1)
- ☐ Bell pepper, green (1)

- ☐ Bell pepper, yellow (1)
- ☐ Bell peppers, red (2)
- ☐ Broccoli coleslaw (1 cup)
- ☐ Butternut squash (1½ cups, cubed)
- ☐ Carrots, cut into chip shapes (¾ cup)
- ☐ Carrots, shredded (½ cup)
- ☐ Celery (2 stalks)
- ☐ Cherry tomatoes (½ cup)
- ☐ Cucumber (¾ cup, sliced)
- ☐ Green onions (4)
- ☐ Green spring salad mix (3 cups)
- ☐ Jalapeño pepper (1)
- ☐ Parsnips (2)
- ☐ Plum tomato (1)
- ☐ Poblano peppers (2)
- ☐ Romaine lettuce (1 cup)

Nuts, Seeds, and Miscellaneous

- ☐ 100 percent all-fruit raspberry jam (2 teaspoons)
- ☐ Agave nectar (2 teaspoons)
- ☐ Almonds (1 tablespoon sliced)
- ☐ Candied ginger (about 3 tablespoons, chopped)
- ☐ Crepe shell, ready made and unfilled (1)
- ☐ Dill pickles (3 slices)
- ☐ Hazelnuts (1 tablespoon, chopped)
- ☐ Hot sauce (1 to 2 dashes)
- ☐ Light beer (12-ounce bottle)
- ☐ Mayonnaise, light canola (1 tablespoon)
- ☐ Peanuts (10 in shell)
- ☐ Pecans (about 2 tablespoons, chopped)
- ☐ Tortilla chips, whole grain (7 chips)

Refrigerated Products

- ☐ Cheddar cheese (2 tablespoons, shredded)
- ☐ Cottage cheese, low fat (¾ cup)
- ☐ Eggs (3 whole + 6 whites)
- ☐ Mozzarella cheese, part skim (2 tablespoons, shredded)
- ☐ Plain yogurt, low fat (2 6-ounce containers)

- ☐ Sour cream, low fat (2 tablespoons)
- ☐ Tempeh (2 ounces from 8-ounce package)
- ☐ Tofu, extra firm (½ cup)

Canned and Frozen Goods

Artichoke hearts, canned in water (½ cup)

- ☐ Black beans, canned (1¼ cups)
- ☐ Cannellini beans, canned (¾ cup)
- ☐ Corn, canned no-salt-added (¼ cup)
- ☐ Garbanzo beans, canned (1½ cups)
- ☐ Great Northern beans, canned (½ cup)
- ☐ Navy beans, canned (½ cup)
- ☐ Pineapple rings, canned in own juice (3 rings)
- ☐ Pinto beans, canned (1½ cups)
- ☐ Pumpkin, canned (¼ cup)
- ☐ Refried black beans, canned low-fat (⅓ cup)
- ☐ Frozen edamame, or shelled green soybeans (½ cup)
- ☐ Frozen mixed berries, unsweetened (¾ cup)
- ☐ Frozen stir-fry mixed vegetables (2 cups)
- ☐ Frozen waffles, whole grain (2)
- ☐ Vegetarian "chicken" patty (1)
- ☐ Veggie burger, black bean (1)

Week Five Recipes, Meal Plan, Shopping List

Week Five Flex Breakfasts

Cottage Cheese with Melon and Fresh Mint

Mint is an herb that I will only use fresh; the dried version doesn't have much flavor. Mint has medicinal properties that may help with digestion and bloating. Put mint leaves in water or club soda for a refreshing, lightly flavored beverage.

1 cup low-fat cottage cheese
1½ cups chopped cantaloupe and honeydew
3 tablespoons chopped fresh mint
2 teaspoons agave nectar

Top cottage cheese with melon, mint, and a drizzle of agave nectar.

292 calories, 3 g total fat, 2 g saturated fat, 9 mg cholesterol, 72 mg sodium, 39 g carbohydrates, 2 g fiber, 30 g protein

Dried Cherry and Pistachio Oatmeal

A trendy breakfast spot in Chicago called Milk and Honey Cafe serves wonderful oatmeal with plump, tart dried cherries and walnuts—but I like pistachios in this even more.

½ cup water
½ cup skim milk or soy milk
½ cup rolled oats
2 tablespoons dried cherries
1 tablespoon chopped pistachios
1 teaspoon maple syrup

Bring water, milk, and oats to a boil. Simmer and stir for 5 minutes. Top with cherries, pistachios, and syrup.

300 calories, 6 g total fat, 1 g saturated fat, 2 mg cholesterol, 61 mg sodium, 51 g carbohydrates, 6 g fiber, 13 g protein

Spicy Breakfast Burrito

This Mexican breakfast can be made in about 5 minutes, or make a big batch on the weekend, freeze it, and microwave one for a fast breakfast on the go.

1 whole egg + 2 egg whites
¼ cup canned black beans, rinsed and drained
2 tablespoons canned chopped green chilies
2 tablespoons shredded cheddar cheese
Cooking spray
1 small (6-inch) whole-grain tortilla

Mix eggs, beans, chilies, and cheese together and then scramble mixture in pan sprayed with cooking spray over medium heat. Wrap in tortilla.

304 calories, 11 g total fat, 5 g saturated fat, 226 mg cholesterol, 509 mg sodium, 33 g carbohydrates, 5 g fiber, 24 g protein

Flex Swap 1 whole egg + 2 egg whites with ½ cup crumbled firm tofu sauteéd with ⅛ teaspoon turmeric (for yellow color).

Vanilla-Berry Smoothie

This is a refreshing smoothie—if you would like it really thick and cold, use unthawed frozen berries.

1½ cup (12 ounces) plain low-fat kefir (drinkable yogurt product)
¾ cup unsweetened frozen berries, thawed
1 tablespoon honey
¼ teaspoon vanilla extract

Blend ingredients in blender or with hand blender until smooth.

291 calories, 4 g total fat, 2 g saturated fat, 14 mg cholesterol, 414 mg sodium, 52 g carbohydrates, 6 g fiber, 14 g protein

Waffles with Cinnamon-Spice Apple Compote

This recipe tastes like apple-pie waffles.

1 apple, diced
½ teaspoon pie spice (apple or pumpkin)
1 teaspoon maple syrup
2 frozen whole-grain waffles, toasted

In covered pot over medium heat, simmer apple, spice, and maple syrup for 5 minutes until apple is tender. Top toasted waffles with apple compote.

289 calories, 9 g total fat, 2 g saturated fat, 70 mg cholesterol, 369 mg sodium, 49 g carbohydrates, 5 g fiber, 7 g protein

Double Corn Pancakes with Maple Syrup and Berries

I rarely specify brands, but I am gaga over Arrowhead Mills multigrain pancake mix. The first ingredient is whole-grain yellow corn, and it also has whole wheat, brown rice, and whole rye. You just add water and oil.

- 1/3 cup *prepared* whole-grain pancake mix (such as Arrowhead Mills, Bob's Red Mill, or Krusteaz)
- 1/4 cup canned no-salt-added corn, drained
- Cooking spray
- 2 teaspoons maple syrup
- 1/2 cup unsweetened mixed berries (fresh or thawed frozen)

Mix batter and corn. Cook about three 4-inch pancakes over low-medium heat on skillet sprayed with cooking spray. Top with syrup and berries.

291 calories, 10 g total fat, 2 g saturated fat, 47 mg cholesterol, 398 mg sodium, 48 g carbohydrates, 7 g fiber, 8 g protein

Veggie Hash and Sausage

Potatoes are not the only vegetable that work well grated and panfried as hash browns. This is a "grate" way to add more veggies to your morning meal.

- 2 teaspoons olive oil
- 2 cups *grated* mixed vegetables: potato, onion, zucchini, eggplant
- ½ cup vegetarian sausage-style crumbles
- 1 tablespoon Italian seasoning
- ½ teaspoon smoky paprika

Heat oil in skillet. Toss together shredded vegetables, crumbles, Italian seasoning, and paprika. Put vegetable mixture in skillet, and cook over medium heat for 6 to 8 minutes (without stirring) on first side; then flip to cook the other side another 6 to 8 minutes.

294 calories, 12 g total fat, 2 g saturated fat, 0 mg cholesterol, 250 mg sodium, 35 g carbohydrates, 9 g fiber, 15 g protein

Flex Swap ½ cup vegetarian soy crumbles for 2 ounces cooked, diced low-fat chicken sausage.

Week Five Flex Lunches

Beans and Rice with Red Chili Sauce

Beans and rice are a dynamic duo—high in fiber, protein, and flavor. The red chili sauce is so simple and healthy and takes basic beans and rice to a whole new culinary level.

- ¼ onion, chopped
- 1 teaspoon olive oil
- ½ cup no-salt-added tomato sauce
- 2 teaspoons chili powder
- ½ cup canned pinto beans, rinsed, drained, and heated
- ¾ cup cooked brown rice (precooked microwavable or, if time allows, simmer your own)
- ½ small green bell pepper, diced

In a medium pan, sauté onion in olive oil for 3 minutes until tender. Add in tomato sauce and chili powder, and cook an additional 5 minutes. Serve sauce on top of hot beans, cooked rice, and diced green pepper.

413 calories, 8 g total fat, 1 g saturated fat, 0 mg cholesterol, 76 mg sodium, 76 g carbohydrates, 15 g fiber, 14 g protein

Spinach Salad with Pumpkin Seeds and Avocado

This salad has many different shades of green, so I affectionately call this dish the Green Monster.

- 4 cups baby spinach
- 2 tablespoons hulled green pumpkin seeds (pepitas)
- 1/4 avocado, diced
- 3 dried apricots, chopped
- 2 tablespoons Universal Lemon-Flax Vinaigrette (see Index) or low-fat Italian dressing

Toss together all ingredients.

387 calories, 29 g total fat, 4 g saturated fat, 0 mg cholesterol, 140 mg sodium, 26 g carbohydrates, 8 g fiber, 14 g protein

Burger with Feta and Spinach

Feta is a favorite cheese of mine because you need only a small amount to add big flavor. The dill and cucumber salad complete this Greek-style lunch.

- 1 vegetarian burger
- ¾ cup baby spinach
- ½ ounce feta cheese, crumbled
- 1 whole-grain hamburger bun
- 1 cup chopped cucumber
- 1 tablespoon chopped fresh dill
- 2 tablespoons Universal Lemon-Flax Vinaigrette (see Index) or low-fat Italian dressing

Heat burger, top with spinach and feta, and serve on bun. Toss cucumber, dill, and dressing to serve on the side.

401 calories, 21 g total fat, 4 g saturated fat, 13 mg cholesterol, 828 mg sodium, 35 g carbohydrates, 8 g fiber, 22 g protein

Fact Stack

Use the 25-25-50 rule to reportion your meals. Aim to have your plate filled with 25 percent whole grains, such as brown rice or whole-grain pasta; 25 percent lean proteins, such as beans or fish; and 50 percent (or more) of fresh produce!

White Bean and Pesto Pita

Pesto packs a mighty flavor punch, but it also can pack on weight with its high calorie content. It's just too tasty to go without, so just measure carefully.

¾ cup canned Great Northern beans, rinsed and drained
½ cup cherry tomatoes, halved
1 tablespoon prepared pesto
1 whole-grain pita pocket, split in half

Mix beans, tomatoes, and pesto. Stuff mixture into pita halves.

393 calories, 9 g fat, 0 g saturated fat, 0 mg cholesterol, 610 mg sodium, 63 g carbohydrates, 14 g fiber, 20 g protein

Flex Swap ½ cup Great Northern beans for 2 ounces cooked, diced chicken breast.

Cucumber-Hummus Wrap

This is creamy, crunchy, and chewy at the same time and couldn't be easier to make.

- 2 small (6-inch) whole-grain tortillas
- 4 tablespoons hummus
- 1 cup sliced cucumber
- ½ ounce feta cheese, crumbled
- ½ teaspoon smoky paprika
- 1 small pear

Fill tortillas with hummus, cucumber slices, feta, and sprinkle of paprika. Serve with pear on the side.

381 calories, 10 g total fat, 3g saturated fat, 13 mg cholesterol, 717 mg sodium, 76 g carbohydrates, 13 g fiber, 14 g protein

Lunch Nachos

Nachos are on every appetizer menu in America because they are a crowd-pleasing favorite. Skip the naughty nachos full of calories and fat, and whip up this nice and healthy version instead.

20 whole-grain tortilla chips
¾ cup canned low-fat or vegetarian refried beans, heated
¼ cup salsa
2 tablespoons low-fat sour cream
2 tablespoons sliced (canned) black olives

Top chips with hot beans, salsa, sour cream, and olives.

400 calories, 14 g total fat, 3 g saturated fat, 11 mg cholesterol, 623 mg sodium, 57 g carbohydrates, 10 g fiber, 14 g protein

Flex Swap 2 tablespoons dairy-based sour cream for 2 tablespoons of the vegetarian version.

Grilled Cheese and Rosemary-Tomato Sandwich

Rosemary tastes great with any tomato dish. This is a more adult and vegetable-focused version of a classic grilled-cheese sandwich.

- 2 slices whole-grain bread
- 1 slice (1 ounce) part-skim mozzarella
- 2 thick slices tomato
- ½ teaspoon dried rosemary
- Cooking spray
- 1 cup low-sodium black bean soup (brands with less than 500 mg sodium per cup)

Make sandwich with bread, cheese, tomato, and sprinkle of rosemary. Spray outside of sandwich with cooking spray, and grill. Serve with warmed soup.

405 calories, 11 g total fat, 6 g saturated fat, 15 mg cholesterol, 454 mg sodium, 56 g carbohydrates, 5 g fiber, 22 g protein

Flex Swap 1 slice dairy-based mozzarella cheese for 1 slice of a vegetarian mozzarella version.

Week Five Flex Dinners

White Bean Chili

My husband and I love this so much we gave the recipe as a holiday present to family and friends a few years ago!

¼ yellow onion, chopped
1 clove garlic, minced
1 teaspoon Italian seasoning
½ teaspoon ground cumin
1 teaspoon olive oil
1 cup no-salt-added crushed tomatoes (*not* drained)
4 tablespoons green salsa
1 cup water
1 cup canned cannellini beans, drained and rinsed
½ lime, juiced
1 small whole-grain roll

Sauté onion, garlic, Italian seasoning, and cumin in oil over medium heat for 3 minutes. Add tomatoes, salsa, water, and beans, and bring to boil. Simmer 10 minutes, and serve with lime juice on top and whole-grain roll on the side.

501 calories, 11 g total fat, 2 g saturated fat, 1 mg cholesterol, 239 mg sodium, 81 g carbohydrates, 17 g fiber, 24 g protein

Flex Swap ½ cup cannellini beans for 2 ounces cooked, diced chicken breast.

Fried Brown Rice with Asparagus and Almonds

The "fried" rice is actually just lightly sautéed. Chopping the garbanzo beans adds a great texture. This is a favorite in my cooking classes.

- 1 teaspoon sesame oil
- 2 tablespoons rice vinegar
- 1 clove garlic, minced
- ½-inch chunk ginger, grated
- 8 asparagus spears, cut diagonally into 1-inch pieces
- ¾ cup cooked brown rice (precooked microwavable or, if time allows, simmer your own)
- ½ cup canned garbanzo beans, rinsed, drained, and chopped
- 2 tablespoons slivered almonds, toasted
- 2 green onions, chopped

Sauté oil, vinegar, garlic, ginger, and asparagus over medium heat for 5 minutes. Add cooked rice and chopped beans, and sauté for another 5 to 7 minutes. Top with almonds and green onions.

487 calories, 17 g total fat, 2 g saturated fat, 0 mg cholesterol, 74 mg sodium, 71 g carbohydrates, 14 g fiber, 18 g protein

Vegetable Enchiladas

Simple tomato sauce with a little onion and chili powder is transformed into a fast and flavorful red enchilada sauce.

- 1/4 onion, chopped
- 1/2 cup no-salt-added tomato sauce
- 2 teaspoons chili powder
- 1 teaspoon olive oil
- 1/2 cup canned pinto beans, rinsed and drained
- 1 cup frozen vegetables (broccoli, cauliflower, carrot), warmed and chopped
- 2 small (6-inch) whole-grain tortillas
- 3 tablespoons shredded cheddar cheese

Sauté onion, tomato sauce, and chili powder in oil over medium heat for 7 minutes. Put 1/4 cup tomato-sauce mixture on bottom of small casserole dish. Roll beans and veggies into tortillas, and lay filled tortillas in sauce. Cover both with remaining sauce, and top with cheese. Broil until cheese is bubbly and golden, about 7 to 8 minutes.

504 calories, 14 g total fat, 6 g saturated fat, 22 mg cholesterol, 585 mg sodium, 86 g carbohydrates, 19 g fiber, 24 g protein

Flex Swap 1/2 cup pinto beans with 2 ounces cooked ground extra-lean turkey or sirloin.

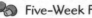

Millet Paella

Smoky paprika, salty olives, earthy black beans, and tender green peas make this a savory dish you will want again and again. If you have them, you can use saffron threads instead of the smoky paprika.

- ½ cup water
- ¼ cup uncooked millet
- 1 tablespoon olive oil
- 1 clove garlic, minced
- ½ teaspoon smoky paprika
- ¼ cup diced jarred (in water) roasted red peppers
- 3 green olives, sliced
- ¾ cup canned black beans, rinsed and drained
- ½ cup frozen peas
- 2 tablespoons chopped fresh parsley

Bring water and millet to a boil. Simmer (covered) for 15 minutes, until water is absorbed. In oil, sauté garlic, paprika, red peppers, olives, beans, and peas over medium heat. Mix with cooked millet, and top with parsley.

498 calories, 9 g total fat, 1 g saturated fat, 0 mg cholesterol, 246 mg sodium, 85 g carbohydrates, 16 g fiber, 22 g protein

Flex Swap ½ cup black beans for 2 ounces (9 medium) frozen cooked shrimp, thawed.

Spinach-and-Mushroom-Stuffed Shells

My first attempt at using tofu was as a replacement for ricotta cheese in lasagna. This recipe calls for stuffing shell-shaped pasta, but the filling can also be used for a big pan of lasagna to feed a larger crowd.

- 2 ounces (about 3) large whole-grain pasta shells
- 2 cloves garlic, minced
- Dash crushed red pepper flakes
- 1 cup raw button mushrooms, chopped
- 1 teaspoon olive oil
- 2 cups baby spinach
- ½ cup firm tofu, mashed like ricotta cheese
- ¾ cup spaghetti sauce (brands less than 80 calories per ½ cup), heated

Cook pasta al dente according to package directions. Sauté garlic, red pepper flakes, and mushrooms in oil over medium heat for 7 minutes. Mix in spinach and tofu, and heat for 3 minutes more. Stuff hot tofu mixture into cooked shells (they will be overstuffed). Top stuffed shells with heated spaghetti sauce.

482 calories, 17 g total fat, 2 g saturated fat, 0 mg cholesterol, 343 mg sodium, 65 g carbohydrates, 6 g fiber, 28 g protein

Fettuccine Florentine with Lemon-Garlic Butter

The light, lemony sauce and the basil make this a very fresh-flavored pasta dish. The trick for the best-tasting spinach is to only lightly wilt it instead of cooking it until it's totally limp: heat the pan, turn off the heat, and quickly just toss the spinach around in the hot pan.

2 ounces (dime's circumference) whole-grain fettuccine, uncooked
1 tablespoon trans-fat-free margarine
1 lemon, juiced
2 cloves garlic, minced
¼ cup chopped fresh basil
3 cups chopped baby spinach, wilted
3 tablespoons pine nuts, toasted

Cook pasta al dente according to package directions. Heat margarine, lemon juice, and garlic in a nonstick skillet over low heat. Take off from heat, and toss together with hot noodles, fresh basil, spinach, and pine nuts.

501 calories, 28 g total fat, 4 g saturated fat, 0 mg cholesterol, 169 mg sodium, 56 g carbohydrates, 4 g fiber, 15 g protein

Orzo with Cilantro-Lime Pesto

This dish is a hands-down favorite in my cooking classes. I have received many thank-you e-mails for this one.

- ¼ cup (2 ounces) uncooked whole-grain orzo (rice-shaped pasta)
- 1 cup fresh cilantro
- 1 lime, juiced
- 1 teaspoon olive oil
- 1 tablespoon pine nuts
- 1 clove garlic, minced
- ½ cup canned black beans, rinsed and drained
- ¼ cup drained and chopped jarred (in water) roasted red peppers
- ¼ cup canned no-salt-added corn, drained

Cook orzo according to package directions. With the chopper attachment of hand blender or in food processor, puree cilantro, lime juice, oil, pine nuts, and garlic to make cilantro pesto. Toss cooked orzo with cilantro pesto and remaining ingredients.

491 calories, 12 g total fat, 1 g saturated fat, 0 mg cholesterol, 41 mg sodium, 84 g carbohydrates, 13 g fiber, 20 g protein

Flex Swap ½ cup black beans for a 2-ounce piece of cooked salmon, tuna, or other fish.

Week Five Flex Snacks and Desserts

Cinnamon-Spice-Crunch Popcorn

The naturally sweet taste of cinnamon complements the bite of chili powder.

- 2 tablespoons popcorn (or 1 100-calorie minibag of microwave popcorn)
- Cooking spray
- 2 teaspoons cinnamon
- ¼ teaspoon chili powder
- 1 tablespoon soy nuts

Pop corn, spray with cooking spray, sprinkle with spices, and toss with soy nuts.

149 calories, 3 g total fat, 0 g saturated fat, 0 mg cholesterol, 13 mg sodium, 28 g carbohydrates, 8 g fiber, 6 g protein

Note: For the most natural popcorn, put popcorn kernels in a plain brown lunch bag and fold open end over three to four times tightly. Microwave for about 2 to 3 minutes (until pops are about 5 seconds apart).

Peapods and Ranch

Veggies like being skinny-dipped into this calorie-conscious, low-fat ranch dip. Packets of ranch seasoning are sold in grocery stores, but I like to get my ranch seasoning from specialty stores (such as penzeys.com or thespicehouse.com) because they are MSG (monosodium glutamate) free.

1 teaspoon ranch seasoning
¼ cup low-fat sour cream
1½ cups peapods

Mix seasoning and sour cream together, and let sit 10 minutes for flavor to develop. Serve dip with peapods.

127 calories, 7 g total fat, 4 g saturated fat, 22 mg cholesterol, 49 mg sodium, 12 g carbohydrates, 2 g fiber, 5 g protein

Wine and Edamame

If you don't drink alcohol, triple your serving of edamame and have water or club soda to drink.

- 5 ounces wine (red or white)
- 15 in-pod edamame (1/4 cup shelled)
- Dash of salt

Heat edamame, and add salt.

153 calories, 2 g total fat, 0 g saturated fat, 0 mg cholesterol, 164 mg sodium, 7 g carbohydrates, 2 g fiber, 4 g protein

Out and About

Pick only one entrée add-on. If you typically order an appetizer, alcoholic drinks, *and* dessert, pick only your favorite *one* to accompany your main-dish entrée.

Cracked-Pepper-and-Salt Pita Chips

Making your own pita chips seasoned with salt and black pepper couldn't be easier, and they taste like you went through a lot of trouble.

1 whole-grain pita pocket
½ teaspoon olive oil
Dash of cracked black pepper and salt

Preheat oven to 350°F. Brush pita with oil, cut into 6 to 8 triangles, and sprinkle with salt and black pepper. Bake on cookie sheet for 8 to 10 minutes until golden and crunchy.

139 calories, 3 g total fat, 0 g saturated fat, 0 mg cholesterol, 326 mg sodium, 25 g carbohydrates, 5 g fiber, 5 g protein

Honey Café au Lait

If you don't make this at home, you can order a café latte at a local coffee shop instead—just be sure to ask for a small size with skim or soy milk. A latte uses espresso, whereas an au lait uses standard brewed coffee.

12 ounces skim or soy milk
8 ounces hot brewed coffee
1 teaspoon honey

Heat milk in pan or microwave, and remove from heat just before boiling to avoid scalding milk. Add 8 ounces hot brewed coffee, and stir in honey.

148 calories, 0 g total fat, 0 g saturated fat, 7 mg cholesterol, 159 mg sodium, 24 g carbohydrates, 0 g fiber, 13 g protein

Puffed Mochi Squares

This is too fun to miss—it is worth the trouble of finding mochi. Mochi (MO-chee) is made from sticky brown rice that is steamed, mashed, and pressed into flat sheets. When you cut the sheets into squares and pop them into a 450°F oven for 8 minutes, they puff up into chewy, little, sweet rice bites with a crispy crust. Make sure you use opened mochi within ten days.

1½ ounces (4 small squares) mochi (Grainaissance)
1 teaspoon agave nectar

Preheat oven to 450°F. Cut four 1-inch squares of mochi. (Note: a 12.5-ounce package makes 30 1-inch squares.) Place on cookie sheet, and bake for 8 to 10 minutes, until they puff. Drizzle agave nectar on hot, puffed mochi squares.

140 calories, 1 g total fat, 0 g saturated fat, 0 mg cholesterol, 35 mg sodium, 30 g carbohydrates, 3 g fiber, 2 g protein

Ginger Bark

This is a healthy way to indulge—ginger is a natural digestive aid, and dark chocolate is good for your heart. You can melt the chocolate in a matter of 20 seconds in the microwave or in a double boiler (bowl sitting over a pot of boiling water). This can be made in bigger batches, put in a pretty tin, and given as a gift!

2 tablespoons dark chocolate chips
1 tablespoon chopped candied ginger

Melt chocolate in microwave or double boiler, and pour on wax paper. Sprinkle ginger pieces into melted chocolate, and refrigerate about 10 minutes until set.

152 calories, 7 g total fat, 4 g saturated fat, 0 mg cholesterol, 3 mg sodium, 26 g carbohydrates, 1 g fiber, 1 g protein

Time Crunch

Make a cooking binder. Organize your favorite recipes from cookbooks, friends, websites, and magazines in a binder. Look through it every week before grocery shopping to inspire your weekly meal planning.

Week Five Flex Shopping List

Make sure you have your fridge, pantry, and spice rack staples stocked (pages 79–80). Amounts in parentheses indicate how much you will use this week.

This list is for one person; multiply the ingredients if you are cooking for more. Check off what you need from the grocery store this week.

Grains

- ☐ Bread, whole grain (2 slices)
- ☐ Bread roll, whole grain (1)
- ☐ Brown rice (1½ cups precooked microwavable or about ½ cup uncooked)
- ☐ Fettuccine, whole grain (2 ounces)
- ☐ Hamburger bun, whole grain (1)
- ☐ Millet (¼ cup uncooked)
- ☐ Mochi or pressed sweet brown rice (1½ ounces, Grainaissance brand)
- ☐ Oats, rolled (½ cup)
- ☐ Orzo, whole-grain (¼ cup uncooked = 2 ounces uncooked)
- ☐ Pancake mix, whole-grain
- ☐ Pasta shells, large and whole grain (3 large = 2 ounces uncooked)
- ☐ Pita pockets, whole grain (2)
- ☐ Popcorn (1 microwavable 100-calorie minibag or 2 tablespoons popcorn)
- ☐ Tortillas, whole grain (5 small)

Fruit

- ☐ Apple (1)
- ☐ Apricots, dried (3)
- ☐ Avocado (1)
- ☐ Cantaloupe (¾ cup, cubed)
- ☐ Cherries, dried (2 tablespoons)
- ☐ Honeydew (¾ cup, cubed)
- ☐ Pear (1)

Fresh Herbs and Flavorings

- ☐ Basil, fresh (¼ cup)
- ☐ Cilantro, fresh (1 cup)
- ☐ Dill, fresh (1 tablespoon)
- ☐ Ginger, fresh (½-inch chunk)
- ☐ Mint, fresh (3 tablespoons)
- ☐ Parsley, fresh (2 tablespoons)

Vegetables

- ☐ Asparagus (8 spears)
- ☐ Baby spinach (10 cups)
- ☐ Bell pepper, green (½)
- ☐ Button mushrooms (1 cup, chopped)
- ☐ Cherry tomatoes (½ cup)
- ☐ Cucumber (2 cups, sliced)
- ☐ Eggplant (½ cup, shredded)
- ☐ Green onions (2)
- ☐ Peapods (1½ cups)
- ☐ Potato (½ cup, shredded)
- ☐ Tomato (1)
- ☐ Zucchini (½ cup, shredded)

Nuts, Seeds, and Miscellaneous

- ☐ Agave nectar (3 teaspoons)
- ☐ Almonds (2 tablespoons, sliced)
- ☐ Candied ginger (1 tablespoon)
- ☐ Coffee (8 ounces brewed)
- ☐ Dark chocolate chips, semisweet (2 tablespoons)
- ☐ Pine nuts (4 tablespoons)
- ☐ Pistachios (1 tablespoon, chopped)
- ☐ Prepared pesto (1 tablespoon)
- ☐ Pumpkin seeds, green and hulled, or pepitas (2 tablespoons)
- ☐ Soy nuts (1 tablespoon)
- ☐ Tortilla chips, whole grain (20 chips)
- ☐ Wine (5 ounces)

Refrigerated Products

- ☐ Cheddar cheese (5 tablespoons, shredded)
- ☐ Cottage cheese, low fat (1 cup)
- ☐ Eggs (1 whole + 2 whites)
- ☐ Feta cheese (1 ounce)
- ☐ Hummus (4 tablespoons)
- ☐ Kefir, plain, low fat (1½ cups)
- ☐ Margarine, trans fat free (1 tablespoon)
- ☐ Mozzarella cheese, part skim (1 slice)
- ☐ Sour cream, low fat (about ½ cup)
- ☐ Tofu, firm (½ cup)

Canned and Frozen Goods

- ☐ Black beans, canned (1½ cup)
- ☐ Black bean soup, low sodium (1 cup)
- ☐ Black olives, canned (2 tablespoons, sliced)
- ☐ Cannellini beans, canned (1 cup)
- ☐ Corn, canned no-salt-added (½ cup)
- ☐ Garbanzo beans, canned (½ cup)
- ☐ Great Northern beans, canned (¾ cup)
- ☐ Green chilies, canned (2 tablespoons, chopped)
- ☐ Green olives, jarred (3 olives)
- ☐ Pinto beans, canned (1 cup)
- ☐ Refried beans, canned low-fat or vegetarian (¾ cup)
- ☐ Roasted red peppers, jarred in water (½ cup)
- ☐ Spaghetti sauce, less than 80 calories per ½ cup (¾ cup)
- ☐ Frozen edamame pods, or green soybeans in pod (15 pods)
- ☐ Frozen mixed berries, unsweetened (1½ cups)
- ☐ Frozen peas (½ cup)
- ☐ Frozen vegetables, such as broccoli, cauliflower, and carrot (1 cup)
- ☐ Frozen waffles, whole grain (2)
- ☐ Vegetarian sausage-style crumbles (½ cup)
- ☐ Veggie burger (1 burger)

Flex Fundamentals: Part Three Summary

- Each recipe makes one serving but can easily be multiplied to feed a crowd.
- Eat breakfast, lunch, dinner, and two snacks each day for 1,500 total daily calories. This is a reasonable starting point for most people. However, depending on activity level, gender, height, and weight you may need to eat more or fewer calories.
- If you are losing weight too slowly, pay more attention to portions. If you are losing weight too fast or are too hungry, add an extra snack or double your breakfast portion (from 300 to 600 calories).
- Mix and match your favorite recipes for a truly personalized flexitarian experience. Each of the thirty-five breakfasts are 300 calories, so you can pick and choose those that most please your palate. The same is true with the interchangeable 400-calorie lunches, 500-calorie dinners, and 150-calorie snacks (choose two snacks per day).
- Most of the recipes include a Flex Swap option for easy ingredient substitutions.
- If experimenting with all of the new recipes each week is sucking your time and energy, look over a specific week and try just one or two of your favorite breakfasts, two or three lunches, two or three dinners, and two different snacks.
- The recipes are quick because they have only five main ingredients and are prepared using fast cooking methods. Keep in mind that the second time you prepare a recipe will be even faster! Additionally, the shopping lists organize your ingredients to save you time in the grocery store (visit dawnjacksonblatner.com to print the lists, or photocopy them out of the book to bring with you).
- Feel good knowing that the nutrition information has been analyzed for you. Each recipe makes a jumbo, no-skimp serving size yet is still calorie-controlled, meets the American Heart Association's main-dish or main-meal criteria for saturated fat and sodium levels, is full of fiber, and contains no artificial ingredients such as trans fat or sugar substitutes.
- Flexitarian food is healthy in a hurry and tastes great.

Part Four

Five Flex Fitness Factors

When I review diet books for clients and the media, one of the criteria I look for is whether the diet book goes beyond just food advice. All *good* diet books should have a balanced, healthful meal plan that has quick, delicious recipes and neither excludes food groups nor pushes pills and supplements. But a *great* diet and lifestyle book should also focus on the big picture of optimal health by including realistic advice on fitness, mental wellness, everyday food issues, cravings, and real-life events such as parties, dining out, and travel and vacations.

Throughout the book you have already seen five different categories of FlexLife troubleshooters: *Fact Stack* troubleshooters answer frequently asked questions about flexitarianism, dieting, and weight loss; *Time Crunch* troubleshooters make healthy changes more speedy and efficient; *Craving Control* troubleshooters are tips to tame even your most ferocious cravings and emotional eating; *Out and About* troubleshooters cover common diet roadblocks and challenges at restaurants, at parties, and while traveling; and *Feeling Good* troubleshooters focus on mental wellness and healthy attitude adjustments. This part of the book adds to the information from the five FlexLife troubleshooters and focuses on five Flex *fitness factors*:

1. The world as your gym
2. Start-up strategies
3. Maintaining motivation

4. Tools of the trade
5. Beating exercise barriers

The benefits you can expect from regular exercise are exciting: weight loss, increased muscle mass, increased burning of fat, protection against heart disease and stroke, lower cholesterol levels, blood pressure control, decreased risk of type 2 diabetes, increased bone density, immune-system enhancement to fight everything from the common cold to some types of cancer, improved mental focus, skyrocketing energy levels, improved self-image and self-esteem, and decreased depression, anxiety, and stress. Additionally, exercisers live about 1.5 to 3.5 years more than nonexercisers. With all these extraordinary mind and body benefits, it would seem a no-brainer to get moving—but a variety of barriers can prevent starting and sticking with an exercise routine.

According to the American College of Sports Medicine and the American Heart Association, everyone should take part in moderate exercise for thirty minutes a day, five days a week (or intense exercise for twenty minutes, three times a week) and strength train twice a week. But even more important than these official guidelines is the guiding principle of flexitarian fitness: *anything is better than nothing.* This means you can feel proud about and benefit from doing anything active—big or small. It doesn't have to be 60 minutes in a kickboxing class or a three-mile walk to "count." Even an extra five minutes here and there can add up to hours of exercise each year! Small changes can make a big difference.

For any weight-loss or healthy-living plan to work long-term, exercise is essential. It's nonnegotiable. You can expect different results from exercise depending on how much you do. There is a general exercising rule of thumb called "30-60-90." Thirty minutes of activity most days of the week helps prevent diseases without much impact on weight. Sixty minutes most days prevents disease and helps keep your weight stable (no weight gain). Ninety minutes most days leads to disease prevention and weight loss. Congratulate yourself on trying to live a fit flexitarian lifestyle no matter how big or small your exercise achievements—trust that anything is better than nothing, and more is even better.

The World as Your Gym

The foundation of living a fit flexitarian life is to build in *activities of daily living*. These basic unscheduled activities don't make us break a sweat, but they do lead to a more active and healthy lifestyle. So use the world as your gym. Bring groceries in one bag at a time, tighten your butt while you are brushing your teeth, go out shopping instead of shopping online, take out the trash, walk into the gas station to pay instead of paying at the pump, park farther away, change the channel on the television itself instead of using the remote control, wash your own car, and walk to your coworker's office instead of calling on the phone. Little things add up. For example, going up and down stairs for a total of fifteen minutes burns about 105 calories. Doing this daily can help you lose almost ten pounds per year! Take the first step to living a fit life by purposefully adding in daily activities and using the world as your gym.

Feeling Good

Redefine yourself. If you have a mental tape that plays messages such as "I am a sweets or dessert person," or "I am not the exerciser type," you are living a self-fulfilling prophecy. Change how you think about yourself, and your behaviors will follow.

Start-Up Strategies

I see many of my clients suffering from *exercise procrastination*: "I know I should, but I just can't seem to get going." Even the most avid exerciser can fall into exercise funks and get out of a routine for one reason or another. *Note:* if you have a heart condition, chest pain, dizziness, or bone or joint pain; are taking medications for a heart condition; or are concerned about your health, consult a physician before substantially increasing your physical fitness.

The following are start-up strategies to get you into a fitness routine for the first time or back into exercise if you've fallen out of the habit.

- **Ten-minute chunks.** Start with just one ten-minute time chunk three to five times a week. You will naturally want to do more to challenge yourself as time goes on, but start small to establish a routine.
- **Walk.** Walking is the most popular exercise of individuals who lose weight and keep it off successfully. Walking is inexpensive, is convenient, and can be done inside or out depending on the weather and situation.
- **Schedule.** Use your daily calendar or planner and actually write in *exercise* as if it were an appointment. Be consistent and plan it at the *same time each day* to get into a routine. At the beginning, you may even want a phone, computer, or other type of alarm or prompt to remind you of the exercise appointment with yourself.
- **Share.** Tell the important people in your life about your new exercise appointment so they can anticipate the change. Don't feel

Out and About

Use healthy travel tricks. Order a nutritious room-service breakfast of oatmeal, fruit, and nuts; ask for an early wake-up call to add in a workout; have the minibar cleared, or don't take the key; and request a room near the fitness center.

guilty about this—you will be a much happier and healthier mom, dad, worker, wife, husband, and so on when you take time to take care of yourself. Really.

- **Buddy up.** Research shows that if you work with a buddy, you will be about 40 percent more successful at sticking with your healthy behaviors than if you go at it alone. Your buddy can be a nearby family member, coworker, neighbor, dog, or even a friend in another state whom you can talk with over the phone or a virtual buddy from an online community. Healthy behaviors are contagious, so keep connected to people who want to be active and who encourage you to succeed.
- **Mind matters.** If your mind is in the right place, getting into an exercise routine is much easier. Focus your mind and energy on building a healthy habit, not on changing your body. If your focus is only on your body, you likely will get discouraged and won't be able to establish a successful routine. Also, keep motivated *before and during* exercise by reminding yourself about that great feeling of accomplishment you feel *after* you are done.
- **Prevent injury.** Before exercise, include five minutes of light walking to warm up your muscles and stretch. After exercise, include five minutes of light walking to cool down your body temperature and lower your heart rate, and stretch. Websites such as for the American Council on Exercise (acefitness.org) and the American College of Sports Medicine (acsm.org) are good resources for more information on injury prevention.
- **Hydrate.** Hydrate before, during, and after exercise to prevent dehydration. Dehydration can make it feel difficult and uncomfortable to exercise and make you feel hungry. The goal is to drink 8 to 16 ounces of water right *before* exercise, 8 ounces every fifteen to twenty minutes *during* exercise, and about 8 to 16 ounces *after* exercise.
- **Focus on feeling better.** After exercise, you should feel better and more energized than when you started; if you feel worse and tired after you exercise, you are doing something wrong. If you regularly exercise until you feel extra sweaty, tired, and sore, you likely won't want to stick with your draining routine, and you could injure yourself.

Maintaining Motivation

After twelve weeks of doing the same exercise, you will burn about 10 percent fewer calories because your body has become trained and accustomed to the workload. Doing the same exercise over and over also leads to mental boredom and exercise burnout. Moral of the story: *mix it up*—don't suffer from exercise monotony! The following methods maintain motivation to be a long-term successful exerciser and reap extraordinary benefits.

- **Track progress.** In a journal, notebook, or calendar, jot down the days you exercise, what you did, and for how long. Then you can see where you started and how far you've come. On those days you don't feel like exercising, it is very motivating to look back at all of your efforts.
- **Get FIT.** The FIT principle is changing *F*requency, *I*ntensity, or *T*ime. Exercise more days per week, put more effort into exercising, or exercise longer, because injecting change into your fitness life is the key to busting a plateau. Typically, people hit a weight-loss plateau (neither losing nor gaining weight) at about six months on any diet plan, but changing FIT is the ticket out of plateau-ville.
- **Cross train.** Try new activities, because *variety* burns more calories and prevents exercise burnout. If you are currently walking or jogging, try adding weight training, yoga, Pilates, hip-hop, belly dancing, kickboxing, exercise videos, or group classes. To get ideas on how to freshen up your dull exercise routine, ask active friends what exercises they have been doing lately.
- **Event motivation.** Sign up for a community 5K walk or run or a similar type of organized active event. You don't have to be a competitive athletic type to participate in these events. They act as motivation to get you in shape and trained for the big day. Once you are there with hundreds of other active people, you'll find it inspirational. Local events are posted in sports or running shoe stores, in the health section of the newspaper, or on websites such as runningintheusa.com or rrca.org (Road Runners Club of America). You can also sign up for an event in another city and plan a vacation around it.

- **Practice "bibliotherapy."** Read books, magazines, newsletters, and websites to get new exercise ideas and techniques. Flip through magazines, and look at the healthy, active people when you need motivation to exercise.
- **Move to music.** Research shows you will exercise about 13 percent longer if you have your favorite tunes playing. Also consider watching movies or listening to an audiobook to make your exercise time more interesting.

Tools of the Trade

Whether you are looking for fitness *variety* or a little exercise *motivation*, one or two of these gadgets, products, or services may be just what you need.

If the Shoe Fits

A good pair of athletic shoes can make exercise more enjoyable and prevent injury. Good overall fit and arch support of the shoe are most important; color and brand are secondary. Consider the following recommendations for purchasing your next pair of shoes.

- **Go big.** Eighty-five percent of us wear gym shoes that are *too small*! Consider a half to a full size larger than your dress or street shoes. There should be about a half inch between your longest toe and the end of the shoe.
- **Left and right.** Try on *both* shoes, as feet are often of different sizes.
- **Heel hugging.** Find shoes that fit snugly on your heels, to prevent blistering.
- **Test run.** Try out shoes in the store, and ask the salesclerk if you can take a brisk walk down the block to test the shoes on the pavement. Keep the shoes on for about ten minutes to ensure they remain comfortable.
- **Pick proper arch support.** Look at your old shoes to help you determine what kind of arch you have. If you notice wear on the *outside*, you probably have a high arch; wear on the *inside* likely indicates a flat foot or low arch. If you notice an even wear, you most likely have a normal arch.

  If you have a high arch, look for a *cushioned* shoe. If you have a flat foot with a low arch, look for *motion control*. If you have a normal arch, look for a *stability* shoe. When in doubt, ask an experienced salesclerk for help.
- **Replace.** Purchase new shoes every 400 to 500 miles. Expect to get a new pair every four to six months if you are active (walking or exercising 3 to 5 miles most days).

Pedometer

Pedometers are gadgets that count how many steps you do each day. Pedometers may also be able to display distance and calories burned, but they are most accurate for assessing steps and much less accurate for assessing distance and calories burned. You can buy them at any sports store for about $30. Typically, they are clipped onto your waistband and worn for the entire day.

Research shows that people who start wearing a pedometer walk about a mile more every day—seeing the total steps at the end of the day is motivating, and the pedometer acts as a physical reminder to be more active. The goal is to walk 10,000 steps per day, which is about 5 miles or the equivalent to burning about 300 to 400 calories, for most people. When you first get a pedometer, wear it for three to seven days to establish your baseline. Then each subsequent week, aim to increase your number of steps gradually by about 5 to 10 percent. For example, if you find you average 6,000 steps per day, push yourself to walk an additional 300 to 600 steps every day the next week and build from there each week until you get 10,000 steps per day and beyond.

Heart Rate Monitor

This device measures how fast your heart is beating to determine if you are exercising at the right intensity—not too easy and not too hard. It has two parts, a strap and a watch. The strap is worn around your chest up against your skin while you exercise, and the watch displays your heart rate. To quickly calculate the heart-rate range you should be exercising in, subtract your age from 220. Once you get that number, first multiply it by 0.5 (which is the lower end of the range) and then multiply it by 0.8 (which is the upper end of the range). I have found that adding this piece of equipment with heartbeat feedback can breathe a bit of excitement and novelty into a routine rut.

Videos

There are hundreds of different types of exercise videos and DVDs on the market. Videos are offered at a variety of skill and fitness levels. Prices range from about $15 to $40 at collagevideo.com, amazon.com, local bookstores, Wal-Mart, or Target, and videos are also available for rent at local video stores and libraries. They are especially great if you enjoy the convenience of exercising at home, or you can use them in hotels if you travel frequently. You can also consider an exercise video swap among friends, family, or coworkers, as many people have a stash of exercise videos they have grown tired of.

Gym Membership

A gym membership can add variety and motivation to your routine because different equipment, personal trainers, and group classes can be novel and stimulating. Being in a place where other people are exercising and trying creative exercise activities can inspire you and pull you out of a fitness rut. Be sure the gym is conveniently located near your home or office so it is more likely that you will go. *Before* signing your name on the dotted line, *always* ask for a trial week or two to assess how convenient it is for you to use, get a feel for the gym's atmosphere, review the class schedule, determine busy times, and find out if the equipment you want to use is easily accessible.

Personal Trainers

Personal trainers can add fitness variety and face-to-face exercise motivation and accountability. I think they are especially important for demonstrating proper strength-training techniques to avoid injuries. If cost is an issue, try group training with two to five people to split the bill. When choosing a trainer, consider the following:

- **Experience.** How long have they been practicing? What type of clients do they typically see?
- **Certification.** Are they certified by the American College of Sports Medicine (ACSM), the American Council on Exercise (ACE), or the National Strength and Conditioning Association (NSCA)?
- **Education.** Do they have a B.S. or M.S. in exercise physiology or exercise science?
- **References.** Ask for a list of past or current clients.
- **Resources network.** Do they work with other health care professionals. doctors, dietitians, physical therapists?

- **Cost, scheduling, and convenience.** What is the fee per hour? Do they offer package rates? When are they available for appointments. morning, afternoon, evening, weekend? Where do they see clients—at home, at the gym? Do they give couples or group discounts?
- **Personality and gender.** It is important that you feel comfortable with the trainer's style, philosophy, and demeanor.

Home Equipment

There is nothing more convenient than home fitness equipment such as a treadmill, bike, stair-climber, or multistation strength-training gym. Think about your fitness needs and preferences, budget, and space availability, and then start shopping. Investing in high-quality equipment tends to be expensive, but it will be reliable, be enjoyable to use, and last for years. You may find good deals if you buy used equipment under warranty from a reputable dealer. Location is everything—be sure to put the equipment you buy into a space that is welcoming, is comfortable, and preferably has a TV and radio. If you put the equipment in a dark, stuffy, and dreary basement, you won't feel inspired to use it. Most important, before you make the investment, be honest with yourself about how motivated you will be to exercise at home, so the equipment doesn't just turn into a dusty, expensive clothes rack.

Beating Exercise Barriers

If you are struggling to start and stick with a fitness plan, here are common exercise *barriers* and the specific *solutions* to overcoming each obstacle and exercise excuse:

Barrier: Negative self-talk, such as saying any of the following to yourself: "Exercise won't help me," "I have tried before, and it hasn't worked," or "I have so much weight to lose that it won't make a difference."

Solution: Practice positivity. Say motivating things to yourself (even if you don't believe them), such as, "I deserve to be healthy, and exercising is the best way to take good care of my body," or "I am proud of myself for sticking with this healthy habit." Negativity never motivates and will always sabotage your best efforts.

Barrier: Exercise is boring.

Solution:

- **Multitask.** Exercise with a friend and catch up, or watch the news or a movie or listen to an audiobook.
- **Cross train.** Try new activities by checking out local sports leagues, recreation centers, or group exercise classes.
- **Enjoy.** Be sure to choose a variety of activities that you enjoy to keep your interest level up.

Barrier: My family and friends don't exercise and don't support my exercise.

Solution:

- **Invite them.** Tell your friends and family you want to be fit and have fun *with* them. Take a yoga class together, try a rock-climbing lesson, or even plan an active rafting, hiking, or biking weekend getaway.
- **Seek out alternate support.** If you can't find support in your usual places, look in other places such as Internet groups, coworkers, neighbors, people in your fitness classes, or those you meet at local 5K walk or run events. Making new, active friends will help you achieve your fitness goals.

Barrier: I'm too lazy or tired to exercise.

Solution:

- **Force the first step.** A body at rest tends to stay at rest. Force yourself to do something very small such as taking a walk down the street or around the block. Taking the first step is always the most difficult part, but it sparks momentum. In time you will naturally want to walk longer and farther.
- **Work with your nature, not against it.** Plan exercise when you feel most energetic. For example, if you feel most lazy or tired when you get home after work, exercise in the morning or some time before you get home from work.
- **Energize with exercise.** Remind yourself that exercise doesn't make you more tired; it actually refreshes and revitalizes you. It is the best medicine for fighting mental and physical fatigue.

Barrier: I am worried that I will hurt myself exercising.

Solution:

- **Start simple.** Walking is a simple exercise that is safe for most people to do. As you become more confident in your abilities and your fitness level gradually improves, you can add new activities to your routine. If you are concerned about starting a walking routine, talk to your doctor for recommendations.
- **Hire an expert.** Personal trainers can give you personalized tutorials and monitor your movements to ensure you don't get injured.
- **Take a beginner class.** Sign up for a fitness class that says "beginner," because it is designed for people who are new to the activity and the instructor can assess your technique for safety issues.

Barrier: I feel too self-conscious to exercise.

Solution:

- **Solo sweat at home.** Exercise in the comfort and privacy of your home with exercise videos or home exercise equipment.
- **Refocus.** Instead of thinking about how you look as you exercise, think about how strong you are getting, how your stamina is improving, or how your heart is becoming healthier because of your exercise efforts.

Barrier: I don't have time to exercise for thirty minutes a day.

Solution:

- **Short spurts.** It may be hard to find thirty minutes all at once, so squeeze in a few ten-minute bouts of exercise throughout the day. These short spurts will give you the same health benefits as one long workout.
- **Fitness first.** Fit in exercise *before* checking e-mails, returning phone calls, rushing to meet deadlines, and running errands. Once the day's hectic pace takes over, it is hard to break away. Sleep in your exercise clothes or keep them right next to the bed as a reminder.

Barrier: I don't want to have sore muscles or to sweat.

Solution: Go slow and stretch. Exercise shouldn't hurt, so start out slowly and build up gradually to prevent soreness and excessive sweating. Also, be sure to follow your warm-up and cooldown with stretching, to prevent exercise aches.

Barrier: I'm afraid I'll get hungrier if I start exercising.

Solution: Hydrate to decrease hunger. Your appetite should *decrease* immediately following exercise, and if it doesn't, it could be a sign that you are dehydrated. Drink more water before, during, and after exercise to curb your exercise-induced appetite.

Barrier: Walking hurts my knees.

Solution: Sit, swim, and seek supervision. Try doing chair exercises, swimming, or working with a physical therapist or personal trainer to develop a specialized plan that meets your physical needs.

Barrier: It's too hot, cold, or rainy outside.

Solution:

- **Inside workout.** Do indoor exercises using home videos; go to the gym or mall for walking.
- **Dress for success.** Invest in exercise clothes made of special materials that make exercising in bad weather bearable. Look for breathable, sweat-wicking materials to keep you from getting too hot or cold.

Barrier: I don't have enough money to join a gym.

Solution: Find cost-effective exercise options. Check out classes at local park districts, community centers, or hospitals where they tend to be more reasonably priced than at gyms. Purchase or rent home exercise videos, share personal-trainer costs with a friend, or enjoy the most convenient and cost-effective exercise: walking.

Barrier: I am not athletic or the exerciser-type.

Solution: Say no to stereotypes. You absolutely do not have to be a hard-bodied, gym rat to be physically active. Walking is a perfect exercise for someone who doesn't have much exercise experience, because it requires no advanced skills or special coordination.

Barrier: I can't exercise on the weekend or vacation, because I want to relax.

Solution: Redefine relaxation. Start thinking of exercise as a way to relieve stress and to relax instead of considering it a chore. Weekends and vacations that include regular exercise will refresh and rejuvenate you more than just lazy lounging.

Barrier: I can't exercise, because I travel or stay in hotels for business too often.

Solution:

- **Sweats and shoes in the suitcase.** Be sure to pack exercise clothes and shoes for every trip. Also consider bringing exercise DVDs as most hotels have DVD players in the room.
- **Request the right room.** Ask to have a room close to the fitness center, because you will be more likely to use it if it is convenient.
- **Workout wake-up call.** Ask the hotel to provide a wake-up call ten to thirty minutes earlier than usual so you can exercise before all of the business meetings and obligations of the day.

Flex Fundamentals: Part Four Summary

- The most important guiding principle of flexitarian fitness is "*Anything is better than nothing.*" This means you can feel proud about and benefit from doing anything active, big or small. Even small changes can and *do* make a big difference.

Flex Fundamentals: Fitness Factors

- The foundation of living a fit flexitarian life is doing *activities of daily living* (basic unscheduled activities that don't make us break a sweat). Make the world your gym.
- Use start-up strategies such as ten-minute chunks, walking, scheduling, sharing, buddying up, understanding that the mind matters, preventing injury, hydrating, and focusing on feeling better.
- Maintain motivation with tricks such as tracking your progress, getting FIT, cross training, getting motivation from exercise events, using bibliotherapy, moving to music, and using new tools and toys.
- New fitness tools and toys can motivate you and wake up your tired exercise routine. Try well-fitting shoes, a pedometer, a heart rate monitor, videos, a personal trainer, gym membership, and home equipment.
- Seek solutions to exercise barriers instead of letting them get in your way of living a healthy and fit flexitarian life.

For more flexitarian ideas and recipes, or to share your flexitarian success stories, visit dawnjacksonblatner.com.

References

American College of Sports Medicine, American Dietetic Association, and Dietitians of Canada Joint Position Statement: Nutrition and Athletic Performance. *Medicine and Science in Sports and Exercise,* 2000; 2130–2145.

American College of Sports Medicine Position Stand: Exercise and Fluid Replacement. *Medicine and Science in Sports and Exercise,* 2007; 377–390.

American College of Sports Medicine. "Selecting and Effectively Using a Running Shoe." Available at www.acsm.org. Accessed January 14, 2008.

American Dietetic Association and Dietitians of Canada Position Statement: Vegetarian Diets. *Journal of the American Dietetic Association,* 2003; 103: 748–765.

American Dietetic Association Position Paper: Fortification and Nutritional Supplements. *Journal of the American Dietetic Association,* 2005; 105: 1300–1311.

American Dietetic Association Position Statement: Total Diet Approach to Communicating Food and Nutrition Information. *Journal of the American Dietetic Association,* 2002; 102(1): 100–108.

American Heart Association Food Certification Program. Available at www .americanheart.org/presenter.jhtml?identifier=4973. Accessed January 14, 2008.

American Institute for Cancer Research and World Cancer Research Fund. *Food, Nutrition, Physical Activity and the Prevention of Cancer: A Global Perspective,* Second Expert Report 2007. Available at www .dietandcancerreport.org. Accessed on January 14, 2008.

Andrade, A., T. Minaker, and K. Melanson. "Eating Rate and Satiation." *Obesity,* 2006; 14 (Suppl): A6–A7.

Barnard, N. D., J. Cohen, D. J. A. Jenkins, G. Turner-McGrievy, L. Gloede, B. Jaster, K. Seidel, A. A. Green, and S. Talpers. "A Low-Fat Vegan Diet Improves Glycemic Control and Cardiovascular Risk Factors in a Randomized

Clinical Trial in Individuals with Type 2 Diabetes." *Diabetes Care*, 2006; 29: 1777–1783.

Barnard, N. D., A. R. Scialli, G. Turner-McGrievy, A. Lanou, and J. Glass. "The Effects of a Low-Fat Plant-Based Dietary Intervention on Body Weight, Metabolism, and Insulin Sensitivity." *The American Journal of Medicine*, 2005; 118(9): 991–997.

Barr, S. I., and G. E. Chapman. "Perceptions and Practices of Self-Defined Current Vegetarian, Former Vegetarian and Nonvegetarian Women." *Journal of the American Dietetic Association*, 2002; 102(3): 354–360.

Bazzano, L. A., J. He, L. G. Ogden, C. Loria, S. Vupputuri, L. Myers, and P. K. Whelton. "Legume Consumption and Risk of Coronary Heart Disease in U.S. Men and Women: NHANES I Epidemiologic Follow-up Study." *Archives of Internal Medicine*, 2001; 161(21): 2573–2578.

Beck, M. E. "Dinner Preparation in the Modern United States." *British Food Journal*, 2007; 109(7): 531–547.

Bell, K. I., and B. J. Tepper. "Short-Term Vegetable Intake by Young Children Classified by 6-n Prop Bitter Taste Phenotype." *American Journal of Clinical Nutrition*, 2006; 84: 245–251.

Bellisle, F., and A. M. Dalix. "Cognitive Restraint Can Be Offset by Distraction, Leading to Increased Meal Intake in Women." *American Journal of Clinical Nutrition*, 2001; 74(2): 197–200.

Berkow, S. E., and N. D. Barnard. "Blood Pressure Regulation and Vegetarian Diets." *Nutrition Review*, 2005; 63(1): 1–8.

Berkow, S. E., and N. D. Bernard. "Vegetarian Diets and Weight Status." *Nutrition Review*, 2006; 64(4): 175–188.

Bharani, A., A. Sahu, and V. Mathew. "Effect of Passive Distraction on Treadmill Exercise Test Performance in Healthy Males Using Music." *International Journal of Cardiology*, 2004; 97(2): 305–306.

Bish, C. L., H. M. Blanck, M. K. Serdula, M. Marcus, H. W. Kohl III, and L. K. Khan. "Diet and Physical Activity Behaviors Among Americans Trying to Lose Weight: 2000 Behavioral Risk Factor Surveillance System." *Obesity Research*, 2005; 13(3): 596–607.

Bowman, S. A. "Television Viewing Characteristics of Adults: Correlations to Eating Practices and Overweight and Health Status." *Preventing Chronic Disease* [serial online], 2006; 3(2). Available at www.cdc.gov/pcd/issues/2006/apr/05_0139.htm. Accessed on January 14, 2008.

Bravata, D. M., C. Smith-Spangler, V. Sundaram, A. L. Gienger, N. Lin, R. Lewis, C. D. Stave, I. Olkin, and J. R. Sirard. "Using Pedometers to Increase Physical

Activity and Improve Health: A Systematic Review." *Journal of the American Medical Association*, 2007; 298(19): 2296–2304.

Burke, L. E., M. Warziski, M. A. Styn, E. Music, A. G. Hudson, and S. M. Sereika. "A Randomized Clinical Trial of a Standard vs. Vegetarian Diet for Weight Loss: The Impact of Treatment Preference. *International Journal of Obesity*, 2008; 166–176.

Burns, C. M., M. A. Tijhuis, and J. C. Seidell. "The Relationship Between Quality of Life and Perceived Body Weight and Dieting History in Dutch Men and Women." *International Journal of Obesity and Related Metabolic Disorders*, 2001; 25(9): 1386–1392.

Canton, S. J., M. Ball, A. Ahern, and M. M. Hetherington. "Dose-Dependent Effects of Alcohol on Appetite and Food Intake." *Physiology and Behavior*, 2004; 81(1): 51–58.

Casagrande, S. S., Y. Wang, C. Anderson, and T. L. Gary. "Have Americans Increased Their Fruit and Vegetable Intake? The Trends Between 1988–2002." *American Journal of Preventive Medicine*, 2007; 32(4): 257–263.

Cassady, D., J. M. Jetter, and J. Culp. "Is Price a Barrier to Eating More Fruits and Vegetables for Low-Income Families?" *Journal of the American Dietetic Association*, 2007; 107(11): 1909–1915.

Centers for Disease Control. "Trends in Intake of Energy and Macronutrients, U.S. 1971–2000." *Morbidity and Mortality Weekly Report*, 2004; 53: 80–82. Available at www.cdc.gov/MMWR/preview/mmwrhtml/mm5304a3.htm. Accessed on January 14, 2008.

Cho, S. C., M. Dietrich, C. J. P. Brown, C. A. Clark, and G. Block. "The Effect of Breakfast Type on Total Daily Energy Intake and Body Mass Index." *Journal of the American College of Nutrition*, 2003; 22(4): 296–302.

Darmadi-Blackberry, I., M. L. Wahlqvist, A. Kouris-Blazos, B. Steen, W. Lukito, Y. Horie, and K. Horie. "Legumes: The Most Important Dietary Predictor of Survival in Older People of Different Ethnicities." *Asia Pacific Journal of Clinical Nutrition*, 2004; 13(2): 217–220.

Dhingra, R., L. Sullivan, P. F. Jaques, T. J. Wang, C. S. Fox, J. B. Meigs, R. B. D'Agostino, J. M. Gaziano, and R. S. Vasan. "Soft Drink Consumption and Risk of Developing Cardiometabolic Risk Factors and the Metabolic Syndrome in Middle-Aged Adults in the Community." *Circulation*, 2007; 116: 480–488.

Diliberti, N., P. L. Bordi, M. T. Conklin, L. S. Roe, and B. J. Rolls. "Increased Portion Size Leads to Increased Intake in a Restaurant Meal." *Obesity Research*, 2004; 12(3): 562–568.

Drapeau, V., N. King, M. Hetherington, E. Doucet, J. Blundell, and A. Tremblay. "Appetite Sensations and Satiety Quotient: Predictors of Energy Intake and Weight Loss." *Appetite*, 2007; 48: 159–166.

Duyff, R. L. *American Dietetic Association Complete Food and Nutrition Guide.* 3rd ed. Hoboken, NJ: John Wiley & Sons Inc., 2006.

Ello-Martin, J. A., J. H. Ledikwe, and B. J. Rolls. "The Influence of Food Portion Size and Energy Density on Energy Intake: Implications for Weight Management." *American Journal of Clinical Nutrition*, 2005; 82 (1 Suppl): 236S–241S.

Farshchi, H. R., M. A. Taylor, and I. A. Macdonald. "Beneficial Metabolic Effects of Regular Meal Frequency on Dietary Thermogenesis, Insulin Sensitivity, and Fasting Lipid Profiles in Healthy Obese Women." *American Journal of Clinical Nutrition*, 2005; 81: 16–24.

Food and Drug Administration. "Definition of Low Sodium." Available at www.cfsan.fda.gov/~dms/flg-6a.html. Accessed on January 14, 2008.

Forshee, R. A., M. L. Storey, D. B. Allison, W. H. Glinsmann, G. L. Hein, D. R. Lineback, S. A. Miller, T. A. Nicklas, G. A. Weaver, and J. S. White. "A Critical Examination of the Evidence Relating High-Fructose Corn Syrup with Weight Gain." *Critical Reviews in Food Science and Nutrition*, 2007; 47(6): 561–582.

Forslund, H. B., J. S. Torgerson, L. Sjostrom, and A. K. Lindroos. "Snacking Frequency in Relation to Energy Intake and Food Choices in Obese Men and Women Compared to a Reference Population." *International Journal of Obesity*, 2005; 29: 711–719.

Franco, O., C. deLaet, A. Peeters, J. Jonker, J. Mackenbach, and W. Nusselder. "Effects of Physical Activity on Life Expectancy with Cardiovascular Disease." *Archives of Internal Medicine*, 2005; 165: 2355–2360.

Gardner, C. D., A. Coulston, L. Chatterjee, A. Rigby, G. Spiller, and J. W. Farquhar. "The Effect of a Plant-Based Diet on Plasma Lipids in Hypercholesterolemic Adults." *Annals of Internal Medicine*, 2005; 142: 725–733.

Gerstein, D. E., G. Woodward-Lopez, A. E. Evans, K. Kelsey, and A. Drewnowski. "Clarifying Concepts About Macronutrients' Effect on Satiation and Satiety." *Journal of the American Dietetic Association*, 2004; 104: 1151–1153.

Green, A. *Field Guide to Herbs and Spices.* Philadelphia, PA: Quirk Books, 2006.

Green, A. *Field Guide to Produce.* Philadelphia, PA: Quirk Books, 2004.

Guenther, P. M., K. W. Dodd, J. Reedy, and S. M. Krebs-Smith. "Most Americans Eat Much Less than Recommended Amounts of Fruits and Vegetables." *Journal of the American Dietetic Association*, 2006; 106: 1371–1379.

Haddad, E. H., and J. S. Tanzman. "What Do Vegetarians in the United States Eat?" *American Journal of Clinical Nutrition*, 2003; 78(Suppl): 626S–632S.

Haskell, W. L., I. M. Lee, R. R. Pate, K. E. Powell, S. N. Blair, B. A. Franklin, C. A. Macera, G. W. Health, P. D. Thompson, and A. Bauman. "Physical Activity and Public Health. Updated Recommendation for Adults from the American College of Sports Medicine and the American Heart Association." *Medicine and Science in Sports and Exercise*, 2007; 39(8): 1423–1434.

Havlicek, J., and P. Lenochova. "The Effect of Meat Consumption on Body Odor Attractiveness." *Chemical Senses*, 2006; 31(8): 747–752.

Herber, D., and S. Bowerman. "Applying Science to Changing Dietary Patterns." *Journal of Nutrition*, 2001; 131: 3078s–3081s.

Herbst, S. T. *Food Lover's Companion*. 3rd ed. Hauppauge, NY: Barron's Educational Series, Inc., 2001.

Hill, J. O. "Understanding and Addressing the Epidemic of Obesity: An Energy Balance Perspective." *Endocrine Reviews*, 2006; 27(7): 750–761.

Janelle, K. C., S. I. Barr. "Nutrient Intakes and Eating Behavior Scores of Vegetarian and Nonvegetarian Women." *Journal of the American Dietetic Association*, 1995; 95(2): 180–186.

Jenkins, D. J. A., C. W. C. Kendall, A. Marchie, A. L. Jenkins, L. S. A. Augustin, D. S. Ludwig, N. D. Barnard, and J. W. Anderson. "Type 2 Diabetes and the Vegetarian Diet." *American Journal of Clinical Nutrition*, 2003; 78(Suppl): 610S–616S.

John, J. H., and S. Ziebland. "Reported Barriers to Eating More Fruit and Vegetables Before and After Participation in a Randomized Controlled Study." *Health Education Research*, 2004; 19(2): 165–174.

Kant, A. K., and B. I. Graubard. "Secular Trends in Patterns of Self-Reported Food Consumption of Adult Americans: NHANES 1971–1975 to NHANES 1999–2002." *American Journal of Clinical Nutrition*, 2006; 84(5): 1215–1223.

Keim, N. L., M. D. Van Loan, W. F. Horn, T. F. Barbieri, and P. L. Mayclin. "Weight Loss Is Greater with Consumption of Large Morning Meals and Fat-Free Mass Is Preserved with Large Evening Meals in Women on a Controlled Weight Reduction Regimen." *Journal of Nutrition*, 1997; 127: 75–82.

Kerver, J. M., E. J. Yang, S. Obayashi, L. Bianchi, and W. O. Song. "Meal and Snack Patterns Are Associated with Dietary Intake of Energy and Nutrients in U.S. Adults." *Journal of the American Dietetic Association*, 2006; 106: 46–53.

Kruger, J., H. M. Blanck, and C. Gillespie. "Dietary and Physical Activity Behaviors Among Adults Successful at Weight Loss Maintenance." *International Journal of Behavioral Nutrition and Physical Activity*, 2006; 3: 17–27.

Lampe, J. W. "Spicing Up a Vegetarian Diet: Chemopreventive Effects of Phytochemicals." *American Journal of Clinical Nutrition*, 2003; 78(Suppl): 579S–583S.

Lanza, E., T. J. Hartman, P. S. Albert, R. Shields, M. Slattery, B. Caan, E. Paskett, F. F. Iber, J. W. Kikendall, P. Lance, C. Daston, and A. Schatzkin. "High Dry Bean Intake and Reduced Risk of Advanced Colorectal Adenoma Recurrence Among Participants in the Polyp Prevention Trial. *Journal of Nutrition*, 2006; 136(7): 1896–1903.

Lea, E. J., D. Crawford, and A. Worsley. "Public Views of the Benefits and Barriers to the Consumption of a Plant-Based Diet." *European Journal of Clinical Nutrition*, 2006; 60: 828–837.

Ledikwe, J. H., H. M. Blanck, L. K. Khan, M. K. Serdula, J. D. Seymour, B. C. Tohill, and B. J. Rolls. "Dietary Energy Density Is Associated with Energy Intake and Weight Status in U.S. Adults." *American Journal of Clinical Nutrition*, 2006; 83: 1362–1368.

Ledikwe, J. H., J. A. Ello-Martin, and B. J. Rolls. "Portion Size and the Obesity Epidemic." *Journal of Nutrition*, 2005; 135: 905–909.

Loliger, J. "Function and Importance of Glutamate for Savory Foods." *Journal of Nutrition*, 2000; 130: 915S–920S.

Maier, A., C. Chabanet, B. Schaal, S. Issanchou, and P. Leathwood. "Effects of Repeated Exposure on Acceptance of Initially Disliked Vegetables in 7-Month-Old Infants." *Food Quality and Preference*, 2007; 18(8): 1023–1032.

Messina, V., V. Melina, and R. Mangel. "A New Food Guide for North American Vegetarians." *Canadian Journal of Dietetic Practice and Research*, 2003; 64: 82–86.

Morris, M. C., D. A. Evans, C. C. Tangney, J. L. Bienias, and R. S. Wilson. "Associations of Vegetable and Fruit Consumption with Age-Related Cognitive Change." *Neurology*, 2006; 67(8): 1370–1376.

Mushroom Council. Umami. Available at www.mushroomcouncil.com/export/sites/default/foodservice/umamiwhitepaper.pdf. Accessed on January 14, 2008.

National Heart, Lung, and Blood Institute (NHLBI) and North American Association for the Study of Obesity (NAASO). *Practical Guide on the Identification, Evaluation, and Treatment of Overweight and Obesity in Adults.* Bethesda, MD: National Institutes of Health, 2000. NIH Publication number 00-4084, Oct. 2000.

Neumark-Sztainer, D., N. E. Sherwood, S. A. French, and R. W. Jeffery. "Weight Control Behaviors Among Adult Men and Women: Cause for Concern?" *Obesity Research*, 1999; 7(2): 179–188.

Newby, P. K., K. L. Tucker, and A. Wolk. "Risk of Overweight and Obesity Among Semivegetarians, Lactovegetarians, and Vegan Women." *American Journal of Clinical Nutrition*, 2005; 81: 1267–1274.

Nicholson, A. S., M. Sklar, N. D. Barnard, S. Gore, R. Sullivan, and S. Browning. "Toward Improved Management of NIDDM: A Randomized Controlled Pilot Intervention Using a Low-Fat, Vegetarian Diet." *American Journal of Preventive Medicine*, 1999; 29: 87–91.

Nielsen, S. J., and B. M. Popkin. "Patterns and Trends in Food Portions Sizes, 1977–1998." *Journal of the American Medical Association*, 2003; 289(4): 450–453.

Nielsen, S. J., A. M. Siega-Riz, and B. M. Popkin. "Trends in Energy Intake in U.S. Between 1977 and 1996: Similar Shifts Seen Across Age Groups." *Obesity Research*, 2002; 10(5): 370–378.

"Of Interest to You: Who Carries Out Their Meals and Why." *Journal of the American Dietetic Association*, 1998; 98(7): 820.

Otten, J. J., J. P. Hellwig, and C. D. Meyers, eds. *Dietary Reference Intakes: The Essential Guide to Nutrient Requirements*. Washington, D.C.: National Academies Press, 2006.

Ovaskainen, M. L., H. Reinivuo, H. Tapanainen, M. L. Hannila, T. Korhonen, and H. Pakkala. "Snacks as an Element of Energy Intake and Food Consumption." *European Journal of Clinical Nutrition*, 2006; 60(4): 494–501.

Patel, S. R., A. Malhotra, D. P. White, D. J. Gottlieb, and F. B. Hu. "Association Between Reduced Sleep and Weight Gain in Women." *American Journal of Epidemiology*, 2006; 164: 947–954.

Patterson, R. E., A. Kristal, R. Rodabough, B. Caan, L. Lillington, Y. Mossaavar-Rahmani, M. S. Simon, L. Snetselaar, and L. VanHorn. "Changes in Food Sources of Dietary Fat in Response to an Intensive Low-Fat Dietary Intervention: Early Results from the Women's Health Initiative." *Journal of the American Dietetic Association*, 2003; 103(4): 454–460.

Pelchat, M. L., and S. Schaefer. "Dietary Monotony and Food Craving in Young and Elderly Adults." *Physiology and Behavior*, 2000; 68: 353–359.

Pliner, P., and D. Zec. "Meal Schemas During Preload Decreases Subsequent Eating." *Appetite*, 2007; 48: 278–288.

Polivy, J., J. Coleman, and C. P. Herman. "The Effect of Deprivation on Food Cravings and Eating Behavior in Restrained and Unrestrained Eaters." *International Journal of Eating Disorders*, 2005; 38: 301–309.

Produce for Better Health Foundation and the Centers for Disease Control. Available at www.fruitsandveggiesmorematters.org. Accessed on January 14, 2008.

Reinaerts, E., J. de Nooijer, M. Candel, and N. de Vries. "Explaining School Children's Fruit and Vegetable Consumption: The Contributions of Availability, Accessibility, Exposure, Parental Consumption, and Habit in Addition to Psychosocial Factors." *Appetite*, 2007; 48(2): 248–258.

Rizza, R. A., V. L. W. Go, M. M. McMahon, and G. G. Harrison, eds. *Encyclopedia of Foods*. San Diego, CA: Academic Press, 2002.

Rolls, B. J., E. A. Bell, and M. L. Thorwart. "Water Incorporated into a Food but Not Served with a Food Decreases Energy Intake in Lean Women." *American Journal of Clinical Nutrition*, 1999; 70(4): 448–455.

Rolls, B. J., J. A. Ello-Maetin, and B. X. Tohill. "What Can Intervention Studies Tell Us About the Relationship Between Fruit and Vegetable Consumption and Weight Management?" *Nutrition Review*, 2004; 62(1): 1–17.

Rolls, B. J., L. S. Roe, and J. S. Meengs. "Salad and Satiety: Energy Density and Portion Size of a First Course Salad Affect Energy Intake at Lunch." *Journal of the American Dietetic Association*, 2004; 104(10): 1570–1576.

Schyver, T., and C. Smith. "Reported Attitudes and Beliefs Toward Soy Food Consumption of Soy Consumers Versus Nonconsumers in Natural Foods or Mainstream Grocery Stores." *Journal of Nutrition Education and Behavior*, 2005; 37(6): 292–299.

Shintani, T. T., C. K. Hughes, S. Beckman, and H. K. O'Connor. "Obesity and Cardiovascular Risk Intervention Through the Ad Libitum Feeding of Traditional Hawaiian Diet." *American Journal of Clinical Nutrition*, 1991; 53: 1647s–1651s.

Singh, P. N., J. Sabate, and G. E. Fraser. "Does Low Meat Consumption Increase Life Expectancy?" *American Journal of Clinical Nutrition*, 2003; 78(3): 526S–532S.

Sivak, M. "Sleeping More as a Way to Lose Weight." *Obesity Reviews*, 2006; 7(3): 295–296.

Slavin, J. "Whole Grains and Human Health." *Nutrition Research Reviews*, 2004; 17: 99–110.

Smith, C. F., L. E. Burke, and R. R. Wing. "Vegetarian and Weight Loss Diets Among Young Adults." *Obesity Research*, 2000; 8(2): 123–129.

Spencer, E. A., P. N. Appleby, G. K. Davey, and T. J. Ket. "Diet and Body Mass Index in 38,000 EPIC-Oxford Meat-Eaters, Fish-Eaters, Vegetarians and Vegans." *International Journal of Obesity and Related Metabolic Disorders*, 2003; 27(6): 728–734.

Stirling, L. J., and M. R. Yeaomans. "Effect of Exposure to a Forbidden Food on Eating in Restrained and Unrestrained Women." *International Journal of Eating Disorders*, 2004; 35: 59–68.

Stroebele, N., and J. M. De Castro. "Effect of Ambience on Food Intake and Food Choices." *Nutrition*, 2004; 20: 821–838.

Szeto, Y. T., T. C. Kwok, and I. F. Benzie. "Effects of a Long-Term Vegetarian Diet on Biomarkers of Antioxidant Status and Cardiovascular Disease Risk." *Nutrition*, 2004; 20(10): 863–868.

Thorogood, M., J. Mann, P. Appleby, and K. McPherson. "Risk of Death from Cancer and Ischaemic Heart Disease in Meat and Non-Meat Eaters." *British Medical Journal*, 1994; 08: 1667–1670.

USDA Nutrient Database for Standard Reference, Release 14. Available at http://www.nal.usda.gov/fnic/foodcomp/search. Accessed on January 14, 2008.

USDA 2005 Dietary Guidelines. Available at www.mypyramid.gov. Accessed on January 14, 2008.

Van Duyn, M. A. S., and E. Pivonka. "Overview of the Health Benefits of Fruit and Vegetable Consumption for the Dietetic Professional: Selected Literature." *Journal of the American Dietetic Association*, 2000; 100: 1511–1521.

Wansink, B., and Chandon, P. "Meal Size, Not Body Size, Explain Errors in Estimating the Calorie Content of Meals." *Annals of Internal Medicine*, 2006; 145: 326–332.

Wansink, B., J. E. Painter, and Y. K. Lee. "The Office Candy Dish: Proximity's Influence on Estimated and Actual Consumption." *International Journal of Obesity*, 2006; 30(5): 871–875.

Wansink, B., and J. Sobal. "Mindless Eating: The 200 Daily Food Decisions We Overlook." *Environmental Behavior*, 2007; 39(1): 106–123.

Wansink, B., K. van Ittersum, and J. E. Painter. "Ice Cream Illusions Bowls, Spoons, and Self-Served Portion Size." *American Journal of Preventive Medicine*, 2006; 31(3): 240–243.

Wardle, J. "Conditioning Processes and Cue Exposure in the Modification of Excessive Eating." *Addictive Behaviors*, 1990; 15(4): 387–393.

Whole Grain Council. Available at: www.wholegrainscouncil.org. Accessed on January 14, 2008.

Wing, R. R., and J. O. Hill. "Successful Weight Loss Maintenance." *Annual Review of Nutrition*, 2001; 21: 323–341.

Wing, R. R., and R. W. Jeffery. "Benefits of Recruiting Participants with Friends and Increasing Social Support for Weight Loss and Maintenance." *Journal of Consulting and Clinical Psychology*, 1999; 67(1): 132–138.

Wing, R. R., R. W. Jeffery, L. R. Burton, C. Thorson, K. S. Nissinoff, and J. E. Baxter. "Food Provision vs. Structured Meal Plans in the Behavioral

Treatment of Obesity." *International Journal of Obesity and Related Metabolic Disorders*, 1996; 20(1): 56–62.

Wing, R. R., and S. Phelan. "Long-Term Weight Loss Maintenance." *American Journal of Clinical Nutrition*, 2005; 82: 222S–225S.

Wittenberg, M. M. *Good Food*. Freedom, CA: The Crossing Press, 1995.

Wu, X., G. R Beecher, J. M. Holden, D. B. Haytowitz, S. E. Gebhardt, and R. L. Prior. "Lipophilic and Hydrophilic Antioxidant Capacities of Common Foods in the United States." *Journal Agriculture and Food Chemistry*, 2004; 52: 4026–4037.

Young, L. R., and M. Nestle. "Expanding Portion Sizes in the U.S. Marketplace: Implications for Nutrition Counseling." *Journal of the American Dietetic Association*, 2003; 103(2): 231–234.

Zellner, D. A., S. Loaiza, Z. Gonzalez, J. Pita, J. Morales, D. Pecora, and A. Wolf. "Food Selection Changes Under Stress." *Physiology and Behavior*, 2006; 87: 789–793.

Index